HEALTHY CHOICES HEALTHY YOU

BEST FOOD SOURCES FOR 35 ESSENTIAL VITAMINS AND MINERALS

By
Paula C. Henderson

HEALTHY CHOICES HEALTHY YOU
BEST FOOD SOURCES FOR 35 ESSENTIAL VITAMINS AND MINERALS

By Paula C. Henderson

© 2018 Paula C. Henderson

All rights reserved. No portion of this book may be reproduced in any form without permission from the publisher, except as permitted by U.S. copyright law.

ISBN: 9781090221421

For permissions contact:
   paulachenderson@outlook.com
   Cover by Paula C. Henderson

DEDICATION

I want to dedicate this book to my mother for her lifelong example of eating and living a healthy lifestyle. Thank You

DISCLAIMER

THE INFORMATION PROVIDED IN THIS BOOK IS INTENDED FOR YOUR GENERAL KNOWLEDGE ONLY.
IT IS NOT INTENDED AS MEDICAL ADVICE AND SHOULD NOT BE USED AS A SUBSTITUTE FOR PROFESSIONAL MEDICAL ADVICE OR TREATMENT.

Contents

1 ARE YOU NUTRIENT SAVVY? 9
2 MY OWN JOURNEY TO EATING HEALTHY 20
3 FOOD SOURCES: AMINO ACIDS 26
4 FOOD SOURCES: BETA CAROTENE 28
5 FOOD SOURCES: BIOTIN 29
6 FOOD SOURCES: CALCIUM 30
7 FOOD SOURCES: CARBOHYDRATES 31
8 FOOD SOURCES: CHOLINE 33
9 FOOD SOURCES: CHROMIUM 34
10 FOOD SOURCES: COPPER 35
11 FOOD SOURCES: FIBER 36
12 FOOD SOURCES: FLAVONOIDS 38
13 FOOD SOURCES: FOLATE 39
14 FOOD SOURCES: IODINE 40
15 FOOD SOURCES: IRON 41
16 FOOD SOURCES: ISOFLAVONES 42
17 FOOD SOURCES: MAGNESIUM 43
18 FOOD SOURCES: MANGANESE 44
19 FOOD SOURCES: OMEGA-3 45
20 FOOD SOURCES: PANTOTHENIC ACID 47
21 FOOD SOURCES: PHOSPHORUS 48
22 FOOD SOURCES: PHYTOESTROGENS 49
23 FOOD SOURCES: POTASSIUM 50
24 FOOD SOURCES: PROTEIN 52
25 FOOD SOURCES: SELENIUM 54
26 FOOD SOURCES: SODIUM 55
27 FOOD SOURCES: VITAMIN A 60
28 FOOD SOURCES: VITAMIN B1(THIAMIN) 61
29 FOOD SOURCES: VITAMIN B12 64
30 FOOD SOURCES: VITAMIN B2(RIBOFLAVIN) 65
31 FOOD SOURCES: VITAMIN B3(NIACIN) 66
32 FOOD SOURCES: VITAMIN B6 67
33 FOOD SOURCES: VITAMIN C 68
34 FOOD SOURCES: VITAMIN D 69
35 FOOD SOURCES: VITAMIN E 71
36 FOOD SOURCES: VITAMIN K 72

37 FOOD SOURCES: ZINC	74
38 WATER	75
39 UNDERSTANDING HOW FOODS DIGEST	81
44 DAIRY	98
45 NIGHTSHADES	101
46 GLUTEN	104
47 GRAINS	107
48 TOBACCO	108
49 CONSTIPATION	109
50 RESTLESS LEG SYNDROME	110
AND RINGING OF THE EARS	110
51 CANDIDA, YEAST INFECTIONS	111
AND ATHLETES FOOT	111
52 SLEEP	113
53 ARTHRITIS	115
54 HYPOTHYROID	123
55 ALCOHOL	125
56 SOY	126
57 BREATHING CLEAN AIR	128
58 THE IMPORTANCE OF ABSORPTION	130
59 RDA quick glance Table	132
60 HEALTH BENEFITS OF HERBS	137
61 BASIL	138
62 BAY LEAF	140
63 CHIVES	142
64 CILANTRO	143
65 DILL	145
66 LEMONGRASS	146
67 MINT	148
68 OREGANO	149
69 PARSLEY	150
70 ROSEMARY	151
71 SAGE	152
72 TARRAGON	153
73 THYME	154
74 ROOTS AND BULBS	155
75 GARLIC	156
76 GINGER ROOT	157
77 HORSERDISH ROOT	158
78 TURMERIC	159

79 HEALTHY FATS 160
80 HEALTHIEST FOODS BY RANKING 161
81 SUBSTITUTIONS CHART 164
82 EXCEPTIONS 167
83 CREATE YOUR OWN LIST 168
84 GO-TO MEAL FAVORITES 170
85 BANNED FOODS LIST 173
86 STAPLES TO HAVE ON HAND 175
87 INVENTORY AND MEAL IDEAS 182
88 NEW FOODS 186
89 DAILY FRESH FOODS 187
90 BEVERAGES 189
91 START WHERE YOU ARE 190
92 WHEN YOU CHEAT 194
94 HOW THE COUNTDOWN JOURNAL CAN HELP YOU 198
95 CLOSING THOUGHTS 199
96 RECIPES 205
97 BONUS COLORING AND WORD FIND PUZZLE 215
98 REFERENCES AND SOURCES 223
99 ABOUT THE AUTHOR 225

1 ARE YOU NUTRIENT SAVVY?

What's the difference between a vitamin, a mineral, and a nutrient?

Nutrients:

There are six (6) essential nutrients for the human body:

1. Proteins *see chapter 24*
2. Carbohydrates *see chapter 7*
3. Fats *see chapter 79*
4. Vitamins
5. Minerals
6. Water *see chapter 38*

Vitamins and minerals differ in basic ways.

Vitamins are organic and can be broken down by heat, air, or acid. **Vitamins** required by our body to function are:

- Vitamins A
- B1
- B2
- B3
- B6
- B12
- Vitamin C
- Vitamin D
- Vitamin E
- Vitamin K
- Folic Acid (vitamin B9)
- Pantothenic acid (vitamin B5)
- Biotin (vitamin B7).

Minerals are inorganic and hold on to their chemical structure. That means the **minerals** in soil and water easily find their way into your body through the plants, fish, animals, and fluids you consume.

Like vitamins, minerals are substances found in food that your body needs for growth and health. There are two kinds of minerals: macro minerals and trace minerals. Macro minerals are minerals your body needs in larger amounts. They include calcium, phosphorus, magnesium, sodium, potassium, and chloride.

Examples of minerals that are necessary for proper health include

- Calcium
- iodine
- magnesium
- phosphorous
- potassium
- selenium
- sodium
- zinc.

Each mineral plays a different role in maintaining proper health.

According to, WebMD, "minerals are elements that originate in the earth and cannot be made by living organisms. So, as human beings, we need to consume these minerals (either from our diets or supplements) because we are unable to produce them ourselves".

Some of the best sources of minerals are plant-based foods. Plants obtain minerals from the soil, and most of the minerals in our diets come directly from plants or indirectly from animal sources.

If you drink distilled water it is very important that you eat foods that are good sources of these minerals

Intake recommendations for vitamins and other nutrients are provided in the Dietary Reference Intakes (DRIs) developed by the Food and Nutrition Board (FNB) at the Institute of Medicine of the National Academies (formerly National Academy of Sciences).

DRI is the general term for a set of reference values used to plan and assess nutrient intakes of healthy people. When there are no RDAs for a nutrient, the Adequate Intake (AI) is used as a guide. These values, which vary by age and sex, include:

Recommended Dietary Allowance (RDA): average daily level of intake sufficient to meet the nutrient requirements of nearly all (97%–98%) of healthy individuals.

Adequate Intake (AI): established when evidence is insufficient to develop an RDA and is set at a level assumed to ensure nutritional adequacy.

Estimated Average Requirement (EAR): average daily level of intake estimated to meet the requirements of 50% of healthy individuals. It is usually used to assess the adequacy of nutrient intakes in population groups but not individuals.

Tolerable Upper Intake Level (UL): maximum daily intake unlikely to cause adverse health effects.

Abbreviations:

AI...............Adequate Intake
DRIs..............Dietary Reference Intakes
DV...............Daily Value
MCG............micrograms (mcg), sometimes written as ug
MG..............milligrams (mg)
RDA............Recommended Daily Allowance

[There are 1,000 micrograms (**mcg**) in 1 milligram (mg)

(**RDA**) Recommended Dietary Allowance. The amount of each vitamin and mineral needed daily to meet the needs of nearly all healthy people, as determined by the Food and Nutrition Board of the Institute of Medicine.

Adequate Intake (**AI**). An AI is a recommended intake level of certain nutrients based on estimates of how much healthy people need. It's used when there isn't enough data to establish an RDA.

Percent Daily Value. What percentage of the **DV** (daily value) one serving of a food or supplement supplies.

For instance, if the label on a multivitamin (or food product)shows that 30 percent of the DV is provided, you'll need 70 percent from other sources throughout the day to meet the recommended daily goal.

Food Groups

- Vegetables
- Protein
- Fats
- Carbohydrates
- Fruit
- Dairy
- Grains
- Starches

FAQ Answers

Potatoes are in the starches group, not the vegetables.

Legumes are carbohydrates (not true vegetables).
Legumes (beans in the high carbohydrate group) are:

- Chick peas (garbanzo beans (what hummus is made of)
- Black beans
- Lentils
- Kidney beans
- Pinto beans
- Navy beans
- Baked beans
- Northern beans
- Black eyed peas

Legumes are high carb foods to be mindful of if trying to lose weight. If you want to include them in your diet consider increasing your level of activity and daily exercise.

Beans in the vegetable group that are low carb and true vegetables:

- Green beans, Green Peas
- Sugar snap peas and Pea Pods

Your Daily Consumption

The healthiest foods you can consume are low carb vegetables.
They should make up approximately 70% of your daily food intake.
Vegetables have the widest variety of balanced nutrients for the body and many of them are good sources of Protein, Vitamin C, Calcium, and healthy carbs.

Healthy Proteins like meat, fish, and eggs, which are low to no carbs, should make up about 15% of your diet.
Remember that many vegetables offer good sources of protein.

Try for 10% Fat to be included with your diet.
Easily attained when using oils to cook with and when making salad dressings, sauces and general preparation of foods, not to mention good fats like Avocado and nuts. Just remember that nuts are generally high in carbohydrates so eat in limited portions.

Limit pure carbohydrates to about 5% of your diet
and limit that to good healthy choices like a sweet potato, nuts, raw honey, and fruits.

DAILY PERCENT

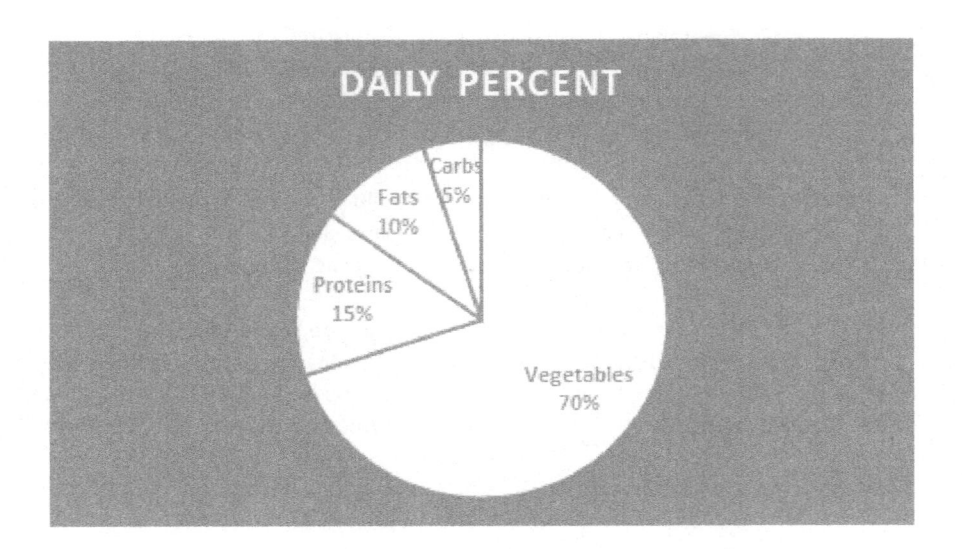

70% Vegetables
15% Proteins
10% Fats
5% Carbohydrates (you will get the rest of your carbs needed from the vegetables you eat)

Throughout this book I will make reference to health issues, conditions and symptoms. They include, but are not limited to:

Excess weight and obesity which I consider a *symptom* of a health issue
Bloating
Gerd and heartburn
Headaches and Migraines
Stiffness
Fatigue and feeling sluggish
Rheumatoid Arthritis
Psoriatic Arthritis
Constipation
Depression
Thyroid disease
IBS
Crohns
Fibromyalgia
Allergies and more!

My personal opinion is that excess weight is a health issue. So anytime I refer to health conditions or symptoms, I am including excess weight. While there are charts telling us what a healthy weight is based on height, age, and gender, I do think those are a mere guide. Only you and your doctor can determine what your heathy weight is.

What we do know, through various studies, is that those of us carrying excess weight are more prone to heart attacks, strokes, diabetes, and high blood pressure to name a few.

Too much fat around our vital organs can interfere with proper function and threaten your health. People who lead more active lives whether through deliberate exercise programs, labor intense careers or just constantly on the move also take deeper breaths bringing in fresh oxygen to all the cells and organs of the body. This is so important and you can read more about that in Chapter 57.

Eating a healthy diet so that you are nourishing your body with necessary nutrients for a body that can function at its best is for everyone. Exercise and leading an active lifestyle will bring fresh air into the body and will exercise the heart muscle even for those who don't need to shed pounds.

Those within a healthy weight range still need vital nutrients, exercise and activity to remain as healthy as possible, maintain flexibility, balance and enjoy a good quality of life as you grow older.

I remember a co-worker who was in a terrible car accident some years back. Her doctor told her she weathered the accident much better than most would have due to the fact that she was in such good physical condition. She was very fit and this not only helped her to escaped more injuries in the accident but helped her to heal much quicker. There are many reasons to be as fit as you can and that won't be the same for all of us as we each have our own challenges and exceptions. Being fit and healthy does not have one look. In the aftermath of Hurricane Katrina there were stories of some of those who drowned. Some, due to being obese were simply unable to physically save themselves. Due to limitations you may not be able to get to a size 8, but I hope that each of you are striving to be the best that you can be!

If you have something that currently works for you, for example, many people eat a bowl of oatmeal every morning and find this keeps them regular. If this is you, continue to do that and only incorporate suggestions from this book that resonate with you for your best health. We are all unique. Oatmeal, as an example, use to work for me prior to my thyroid disease. Now it does not and I avoid it with the exception of perhaps once or twice a month.

> Do these things and I believe
> you will fall at whatever
> your naturally healthy
> weight is for you!

For those of you who do not like deliberate exercise here are some suggestions to create a more active lifestyle:

- Join a community team like softball, bowling, basketball with your city, church or local organizations.
- Take classes like ballroom dance classes
- Join a bird watching group
- Join a hiking group
- Start your own lawn care service on the weekends using a push mower
- Get into the habit of walking the dog or start a dog walking service
- Go dancing on the weekends!
- Join a YMCA and take advantage of the pool, the basketball court and classes.
- Volunteer to pick up trash in your community
- Volunteer for Habit for Humanity and help build a house
- Even if you do formal exercises throughout the week, once a week forego the treadmill and do something fun like one of the activities listed above or make a list of area and nearby parks and each weekend pick a different one to go visit. Walk their trails, and take along a Frisbee!
- Find walking tours in your area for various things. We like to go to all the open houses in our area on the weekends.
- Start riding bikes again!
- Do more around the house:
    o Make your bed every day and change the sheets every weekend
    o Stop using a riding lawn mower and go back to a push mower
    o Wash your windows once a month
    o Sweep the floor and the porch every day
    o Start a big project like cleaning out the garage and stand while going through the boxes rather than sitting.

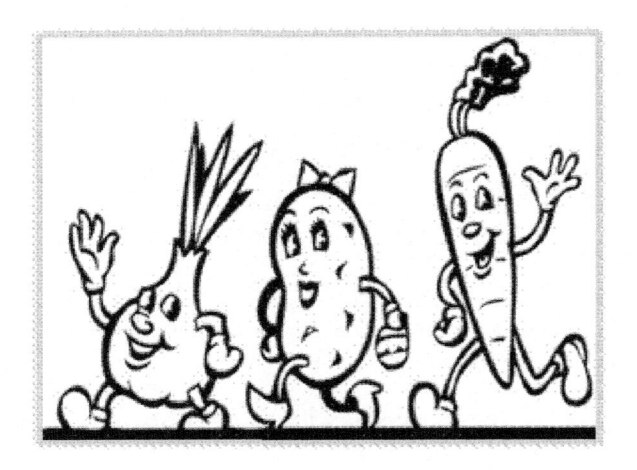

2 MY OWN JOURNEY TO EATING HEALTHY

In 2001 I was just 36 years old. At the time I worked in an office as an Administrative Assistant and started to have problems opening the mail, filing, typing and worse, by the end of the day I was not able to grip the steering wheel of my car well enough to safely drive home.

It was at this time it occurred to me things I had been doing over the past year or so and just dismissed them. The year leading up to not being able to perform my duties at work I had started leaving things on the counter at home so that I would not have to use my hands to open the cupboards to get to everything. I remembered also thinking the plates and glasses were so heavy and started buying plastic to replace them. Why it did not occur to me to question why my dishes suddenly felt heavy I'm not sure except that I was working two jobs and raising my daughter and rarely had time to just stop and think. I was just always moving forward. Thinking about what I had to do next and figuring out how to do that without much question why.

In retrospect I began to have problems in my late twenties but the signs were so subtle and rare that I paid no attention to them. By the time I was 36 and found I could no longer carry on at work I had no choice but to face it and try to find out what was going on.

Doctor, after doctor did not believe me. The most upsetting part of this is that I had no history of feigning illnesses, in fact, I never even got the flu or a cold so I never went to the doctor accept on the rare occasion like for a physical for a job or a tetanus shot. On top of that, not one of the many doctors I saw took any tests to base their decision.

At work they required me to complete a workers compensation form stating that I had been injured at work. I had not been injured at work and told them so and they instructed me to fill out the form anyway so I could receive some benefit payments while I sought medical treatment. I did this, but in doing so I was required to see the doctors they wanted me to see. One was going to rehabilitation for an injury. I explained to the people at rehab who were attempting to get me to do hand exercises that only made things worse. The person in charge of my rehabilitation ask me to lie on the paperwork or they would get in trouble. She explained that she was required to show improvement in her patients after she had worked with them or she would get into trouble. I told her I would not do that as it was not about her. The whole thing became very problematic to say the least and I ended up having to leave work completely without a diagnosis or benefits from anywhere.

The challenge was getting a doctor to at least run some tests to find out what was going on. I saw about eight (8) doctors in Ohio over the course of 2 years and could not get anyone to believe me.

I suspected arthritis and thought a low humidity climate would help and so, after my daughter graduated from high school I moved to the Southwest (Arizona) in 2003.

Backing up to an incident that seemed to trigger even more symptoms. While in Tennessee for my father's illness and subsequent funeral I was walking on a small mountain or large hill near my mother's home, tripping on some roots while at the top I tumbled all the way down making a hard landing on the pavement of a road that wound around and up the mountain. On the way down I bounced over rocks, tree stumps and brush with stickers. While I did not break anything It was after that I noticed problems with my spine, ankles, knees and elbows. All of my joints.

While in Arizona I sought a diagnosis. Moving there in 2003, it still took until 2008 before I finally found a doctor who ran some blood work and did some X-rays and gave me a diagnosis of Rheumatoid Arthritis. That same year I was diagnosed with Hypothyroidism.

Sadly within a year of my diagnosis my husband was transferred to Nevada with his job. I would have to find a new doctor. I wasn't worried at first because I assumed my new doctor would send for my medical records in Arizona. They refused to do that and stated they make their own determinations and I again found myself hopping from doctor to doctor just trying to find one that would run some test. In the meantime I was not getting any medications for health issues.

In 2010 I read an article about nightshades and how they may affect people with arthritis. By this time I was getting weary and very tired and thought well, I'll give it a try. So for a week I did not eat tomatoes. Not noticing any difference I blew it off to myth.

Every year my symptoms worsened and spread. In the years since going off all medications when we moved to Nevada I had grown more and more interested in how diet affects health conditions, triggers and their symptoms.

In my late twenties I had taken classes and became a certified weight loss counselor. I really enjoyed working with the clients and work did not feel like work as I talked all day about something I truly had an interest in.

Now, here in 2012, I decided to take some online classes and read as much as I could about the relationship between one's diet and how it may or may not affect symptoms of arthritis and hypothyroidism. An underactive thyroid also contributes to weight gain and this, coupled with my previous experience as a weight loss counselor really spawned my interest to study this topic thoroughly.

In 2013, after many online courses, reading countless number of research studies that had been done, and talking to hundreds of men and women who had firsthand experience in their own lives, I decided I would try the diet changes again.

This time was definitely different then my first "try" back in 2010. This time I understood clearly what I had done wrong. And this time, armed with all the information I had learned over the past year or so, I was committed to doing it correctly to find out for sure, without a doubt, if a diet change would help me too.

My mistakes in 2010 started with not fully appreciating how inflammation affects the body and not researching how to do an elimination diet the correct way;

1. Eliminating **all** of the foods that are known to cause inflammation
2. Allowing time for what was being stored in my body from the last 30 years to dissipate.

I started a list of all the foods I needed to eliminate for a period of time. The suggested period of time to initially avoid these foods had varying opinions as to how long so I decided on 45 days which I felt would be a happy medium. Looking at the list of foods to avoid was daunting to say the least considering my current diet. I had decided to spend the 45 days gluten free, dairy free, nightshade free, soy free and grain free since they all appeared to contribute to inflammation and some proved to be problematic to thyroid function. I also had to consider low carb since I was having a difficult time maintaining a healthy weight. Looking at it, I realized by eliminating glutens I would be getting rid of most of the high carb foods that probably attributed to my holding onto the weight since being diagnosed with hypothyroidism. All the whole wheat "healthy" foods I had actually added to my diet to try and combat the chronic constipation brought on after my thyroid diagnosis. Which, by the way, had not helped!

I had been chronically constipated for about 8 years even though I had oatmeal for breakfast every morning and had switched to whole wheat breads, brown rice, and other high fiber foods as instructed by a gastroenterologist who last told me he didn't know what else to suggest for me to do. Since doing that I had gained about 25 pounds and was still chronically constipated.

But I digress! So I had made my list of food groups to avoid and as I started to fill in a list of foods within those list it occurred to me that it might be easier to make a list of what was left to eat.

What's left to eat?

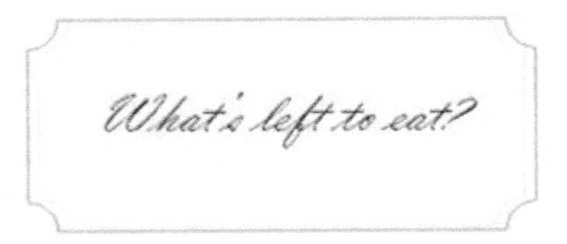

The initial thought of that initially was out of sarcasm but then it seemed, well, yeah! While it is important to know what to avoid, I might find it easier to make a grocery list and create menu's if I have a good list of what I actually can eat. So off to the store I went.

I walked every isle, every department. Making a list of all the foods that were not known to cause inflammation (not gluten, dairy, nightshades or grains) and also no soy foods as it is known to play havoc with the thyroid and your hormones.

As I added more and more foods I found my anxiety start to subside. I realized there were lots of foods I already ate, that I loved, that I could be very satisfied with. Foods I could make familiar meals with.

Back at home I grabbed a wall calendar and started my countdown. Writing 45 on the day I would start. After successfully getting through each day without cheating I would continue my countdown: 45, 44, 43, 42, and so on. I had days I faltered and when I did I started my countdown over the following day:
45, 44, 43, 42, and so on. It took me 9 months of trying on and off before I finally, successfully, went 45 days consecutive. But along the way, during those nine months, I ate much healthier overall and I was eating a lot less carbs. I had lost 33 pounds and yes, I felt 20 years younger. It was wonderful. I was able to do things I had not done in years without experiencing any pain.

Now came time to find out if I could tolerate any of the foods back in my diet without experiencing any symptoms and if so, how much. Yep, another list was started. I knew this time I had to reintroduce foods one at a time over a 3 to 4 day timeframe to see if they triggered any symptoms. I started with raw tomatoes. I did not have to go 3 days though. I had tomatoes for supper and when I woke up the following morning my wrists were quite painful. I chose not to eat them anymore and they were added to my Banned Foods List. I waited for the symptoms that were triggered by the raw tomato to subside (3 full days) and then I tried canned tomatoes. The following day after eating the canned tomatoes I actually felt fine. So I had another serving the second day. And then the third day. It was after the third day I woke up with terrible pain and stiffness. So it seemed I could tolerate one serving of cooked tomatoes every now and then but not within the same week. I have since discovered, through trial and error, my tolerance level for cooked tomatoes is once a month and no more than that.

I used this same process, reintroducing one food at a time.

I get ask the question if it is difficult to not cheat being on such a restricted diet. The answer is no. Not really. I focus on the foods I know I can have that I love, I have found some new foods I had not tried before that are now a part of my diet and the biggest motivation is even though I have thyroid disease I can control my weight and even though I have RA (rheumatoid arthritis) I know how to control my pain without pain medication most days and minimal amounts otherwise. No one wants to live in pain. You feel like you are suffering every day. The problems with the weight gain are also gone. This is my motivation.

3 FOOD SOURCES: AMINO ACIDS

Amino Acids are the building blocks of protein that helps you build and maintain muscle mass.

Muscle plays a central role in whole-body protein metabolism, which is particularly important in the response to stress and the prevention of some chronic diseases.

Both animal and plant proteins are made up of about 20 common amino acids. Of the 20 **amino acids** in your body's proteins, nine are essential to your diet because your cells cannot manufacture them:

- Histidine
- Isoleucine
- Leucine
- Lysine
- Methionine
- Phenylalanine
- Threonine
- Tryptophan
- valine.

Here are some of your Best Sources of Proteins!

- Almonds
- Avocados
- Berries
- Brazil Nuts and Cashews
- Cantaloupe
- Cauliflower
- Chia Seeds
- Green Peas
- Leafy Greens
- Mushrooms
- Olives
- Onions
- Parsley
- Sesame Seeds

4 FOOD SOURCES: BETA CAROTENE

RDA: There is no recommended daily allowance for beta carotene.
The human body converts **beta carotene** into vitamin A (retinol)

We need vitamin A for healthy skin, our immune system, good eye health and vision.

Beta carotene in itself is not an essential nutrient, but once the body turns the beta carotene into Vitamin A, it is essential!

Rich sources of Beta Carotene:

- Apricots
- Asparagus
- Cantaloupe
- Carrots
- Collards
- Fresh Parsley
- Grape Leaves: do a search on your favorite recipe site on how you might incorporate these in the occasional meal!
- Green Peas
- Kale: fresh and frozen chopped kale
- Mustard Greens (leafy green)
- Onions
- Romaine Lettuce
- Spinach
- Sweet Potatoes (high carb food alert)
- Turnip Greens

Knowing the body converts beta carotene into Vitamin A. It should be stated that excess Vitamin A is toxic so supplements are not suggested, but rather sources from food. Talk to your doctor and follow your doctors instructions if they differ from anything else you read here or otherwise for your own health needs.

5 FOOD SOURCES: BIOTIN

Healthy hair, skin and nails.

Also known as Vitamin H

RDA: 30 micrograms daily

Best food sources:

- Almonds
- Avocados
- Cauliflower
- Egg yolks
- Salmon
- Spinach

Biotin is often suggested to those that have been diagnosed with Hypothyroidism. Hypothyroidism can have a terrible side effect on the hair, leaving it dry, brittle, thinning and unmanageable. Biotin is often suggested as a supplement in these cases. It generally takes about one full month before you notice a difference. It is sometimes not noticed until the patient stops taking it for one reason or another and within a week or so starts seeing the damaged and thinning hair return resulting in the patient going back to taking it daily. Start with 5000 mcg per day. If, after one full month you do not see a difference up the dose to 10,000 mcgs per day. Speak with your doctor if you are concerned with taking Biotin as a supplement.

Be sure to also read chapter 58 on the Importance of Absorption. Sometimes the lower dosage is fine so long as you are not hindering the absorption. With a little tweaking many find they can continue to take the lesser dose.

6 FOOD SOURCES: CALCIUM

RDA: Men and Women should both be striving for 1000-1200 mg of calcium per day.

Calcium is a mineral that is necessary for life. In addition to building bones and keeping them healthy, calcium helps our blood clot, keeps your nerves sending messages, and you're muscles contracting.

About 99 percent of the calcium in our bodies is in our bones and teeth. Each day, we lose calcium through our skin, nails, hair, sweat, urine and feces, but our bodies cannot produce new calcium.

It is important to try to get calcium from the food we eat. When we don't get enough calcium for our body's needs, it is taken from our bones.

Best Non-Dairy Sources:

- Almonds
- Bok Choy
- Broccoli
- Chia Seeds
- Kale
- Orange: whole fresh orange. Not juice.
- Sardines
- Salmon
- Sesame Seeds

When choosing Almond Milk in place of dairy milk be sure to choose unflavored original. It has the least amount of sugar and will be much more versatile in the kitchen for sauces and gravies. You can always add vanilla flavoring if using in a smoothie.

7 FOOD SOURCES: CARBOHYDRATES

RDA: How many carbohydrates a person consumes daily is highly dependent on each of our individual needs. Some factors to consider are:

Are you trying to maintain your current weight? Are you trying to lose weight? Do you lead an active lifestyle or a sedentary lifestyle?

An office worker who does not supplement their day with daily exercise will not require as many carbohydrates as a construction worker or a person who runs 3 miles a day.

RDA: The average baseline for carbohydrates is generally 150 grams per day. If you find you need to lose some weight you need to increase your daily activity level and decrease your daily carbohydrate intake to around 100 grams per day. Once you have reached your ideal healthy weight the idea is to only consume the amount of carbohydrates that you use each day. Remember that losing weight is not necessarily about going hungry. If you are hungry you should eat; just choose foods that are low carb and unprocessed. Secondly, learn to stop eating the moment you no longer feel hungry; even when it means leaving one small bite on your plate. And third: Do not eat at all if you are not hungry.

> The most common carbohydrate
> people eat that is
> most often overlooked is sugar.

Sugar, natural or processed, is a carbohydrate. A carbohydrate you should avoid all together if processed, and limit your portions if from a natural, unprocessed source such as fruit or raw honey. Read more about sugar, including the use of Stevia in Chapter 43.

Carbohydrates are the main energy source for the brain. Without carbohydrates, the body could not function properly. Sources include fruits, breads and grains, vegetables and sugars.

A short list of your healthiest and lowest carb vegetables sources are:

- Artichokes Bell Pepper (Nightshade Alert!)
- Asparagus
- Broccoli
- Brussels Sprouts
- Cabbage
- Cauliflower
- Celery
- Cucumbers
- Green Beans
- Kale
- Lettuce: All varieties
- Mushrooms
- Onions
- Radishes
- Spinach
- Tomatoes (nightshade alert!)
- Yellow Squash
- Zucchini

Broth, while not a vegetable, is a low carb companion you can use to make great dishes with your low carb vegetables. Broth based soups, or cream based using the broth instead of milk for soups, sauces and gravies!

8 FOOD SOURCES: CHOLINE

RDA: there is no RDA for Choline, however, a 1998 study showed **AI** (adequate intake) would be on average 550 mg per day.

Choline is an essential nutrient for a healthy metabolism, cell structure and many other complex body functions.

A great article on Choline can be found on ncbi.nlm.nih.gov which is the National Center for Biotechnology

The single best source of Choline is egg yolks.

Aside from that, regular consumption of the following will help to keep Choline in the system:

- Almonds
- Broccoli (cooked)
- Cabbage (cooked)
- Eggs
- Lentils
- Pumpkin Seeds
- Sunflower Seeds

9 FOOD SOURCES: CHROMIUM

AI: In 1989 The National Academy of Sciences established an AI, or Adequate Intake (daily) for the trace minerals. There is no RDA for Chromium.

The **AI**, for an average healthy adult between 19-54 years of age is 25 mcg for women and 35 mcg's for men. [Note this is mcg and not mg]

Chromium supports insulin, regulating your blood sugar.

While traces of chromium are in a wide variety of foods your best sources are:

- Shellfish: mussels and oysters having the highest amount of chromium per serving.
- A fresh, raw pear
- Brazil nuts
- Broccoli
- Garlic

10 FOOD SOURCES: COPPER

RDA: The Recommended Dietary Allowance for adult men and women is 900 mcg/day. Just shy of 1 mg per day.

Copper, a micronutrient, in the diet is necessary for proper maintenance of connective tissue, the kidneys, heart and liver. It also plays a role in your ability to absorb the proper amounts of iron. Copper supports a healthy immune system and has a hand in creating myelin (the sheath covering nerve fibers), collagen (a protein that forms bones, skin, and connective tissue), and melanin (pigment that gives color to hair and skin).

Good Sources of copper:

- Black pepper
- Dark green leafy
- Liver
- Nuts
- Oysters
- Shellfish

11 FOOD SOURCES: FIBER

Fiber, we have learned, is necessary in our diets. We have also learned many have difficulty digesting traditional sources of fiber like whole wheat and whole grain foods. Not to worry! Fiber is also abundant in your vegetables and that will give you the fiber you need without all of the carbohydrates from whole grains. So if you are not losing weight like you thought you would, or, find you are sensitive or even allergic to gluten and grains then you will want to read the list of foods below for great sources of fiber.

RDA: The American Heart Association Eating Plan suggests eating 25 to 30 grams a day from food, not supplements. Some research shows fiber intake among adults in the United States averages about 15 grams a day. That's about half the recommended amount.

Great sources of vegetable, fruit and nut fiber:

- Artichokes
- Almonds, Pecans and walnuts
- Blackberries (fresh only)
- Broccoli
- Brussels Sprouts
- *Flaxseed, ground
- Green Beans (cooked from fresh)
- Green peas
- Raspberries (fresh only)
- Spinach
- Sweet Potato (baked, with the skin) (high carb food alert)

*Ground flaxseed provides your body with the benefits of both soluble and insoluble fibers, whole flax seeds only provides you with insoluble fiber due to its outer shell. Flaxseed is a true plant and not a gluten or grain.

UNDERSTANDING SOLUBLE AND INSOLUBLE FIBER

It is important to consume a balance of foods that are considered Soluble Fiber as well as those that are Insoluble Fiber.

Soluble Fiber is easily dissolved in water and becomes gel-like when it reaches your large intestine so it's more easily broken down by liquids and gastrointestinal fluids and releases certain gases. So be sure to drink water when eating this type of fiber rich foods, and/or combine it with foods that have a high water content.

Insoluble Fiber does not dissolve in water and stays basically intact as it moves through your colon. It absorbs fluid when it reaches your intestinal tract (another reason to be hydrated), which helps other byproducts stick to it, forming the waste you want to get rid of. In the process, it lessens the amount of time food spends in your colon and helps it to exit at the same time. Blockage and constipation are much less of a problem, and bowel movements become much more regular.

Gluten free foods that are good fiber sources:

Soluble Fiber:
- Berries: blackberries, raspberries, strawberries, blueberries.
- Flaxseed, ground or milled
- Oranges (not juice. the actual fruit only)
- Sweet Potatoes (high carb food alert) Try a baked sweet potato for breakfast with butter and a sprinkle of cinnamon.

(tip: berries are the fruits with the least amount of sugars)

Insoluble Fiber:
- almonds, Brazil nuts and walnuts
- avocados
- Broccoli
- Cabbage and Brussels sprouts
- Carrots
- Cauliflower
- Flaxseed, ground or milled
- leafy green vegetables, such as spinach, kale, collards and turnip greens.

12 FOOD SOURCES: FLAVONOIDS

Flavonoids, also known as Vitamin P, provide antioxidant activity in the body. Helping to guard against diabetes, cardiovascular disease and more.

Isoflavones are flavonoids with structural similarities to estrogens

Good sources of flavonoids are:

- Most fresh berries are good sources of flavonoids.

- Green and red vegetables are your best bet for flavonoids:

- Apple
- Artichokes
- Broccoli
- Celery
- Grapes (red and purple varieties)
- Kale
- Leeks
- Okra
- Parsley
- Red Onions
- Red Wine
- Scallions
- Tea: Green, Oolong and Black teas

Thyroid Patients: Just a note to those of you with thyroid disease (hypothyroidism or hyperthyroidism) you may or may not find that these foods affect your thyroid symptoms; either causing them to worsen or lessen their severability. If your thyroid symptoms are not under control with medication try avoiding these foods, much like you do all soy products. Or, if you do not eat these foods as a part of your regular diet you may want to try including them.

I realize this sounds confusing to some but we are all unique and how our bodies respond to foods that have been shown to affect the thyroid can vary greatly in each of us.

13 FOOD SOURCES: FOLATE

Folate is also known as Vitamin B9 and Folic Acid.

Our bodies need folate to make DNA and other genetic material. It is essential to pregnant women and it also may help with depression while also being an antioxidant.

RDA: 400 mcg per day for men and women.

- Asparagus
- Avocado
- Broccoli
- Brussels Sprouts
- Dark green leafy (spinach, kale, collards, swiss chard) *best source*
- Eggs (eat the yolk!)
- Green peas
- Lettuce (all varieties)
- Poultry

14 FOOD SOURCES: IODINE

According to webmd the body needs iodine but cannot make it itself. If you buy salt, always choose a brand marked "with iodine" unless otherwise directed by your physician.

Did you know most iodine is found in the ocean, concentrated from seaweed?

The thyroid gland needs iodine to make hormones. Iodine is not the same as sodium.

RDA: According to the ods.od.nih.gov the average adult needs approximately 150 mcg (not mg, but mcg's) of iodine per day.

Food sources:

- Cod (baked)
- Eggs (whole egg including the yolk)
- Green peas
- Iodized salt
- Seaweed
- Shrimp
- Tuna

Iodine and Sodium are not the same thing. The connection is that the average healthy person should make sure they are using Iodized Salt, which is salt that has iodine added to it during processing.

15 FOOD SOURCES: IRON

RDA: The recommended daily allowance for men is 9 mg per day. For women who are still menstruating the daily allowance is doubled, to 18 mg per day. After menopause, the average, healthy woman should reduce her iron intake to 9 mg per day or as instructed by her physician.

The MayoClinic.org site states:

"Your body absorbs more iron from meat than it does from other sources. If you choose to not eat meat, you may need to increase your intake of iron-rich, plant-based foods to absorb the same amount of iron as does someone who eats meat."

They go on to say that an adequate amount of vitamin C is also needed for proper iron absorption. Stay hydrated too by eating hydrating foods with higher amounts of water content to aide in absorption. Check out Chapter 38 on Water for a list of hydrating foods as well as Chapter 33 on Vitamin C.

Best Sources of Iron:

- Dark Leafy Green like spinach and lettuce varieties
- Green Peas
- Red meat, pork and poultry
- Seafood

Before taking an iron supplement you should always consult your physician. Iron supplementation may cause gastrointestinal irritation, nausea, vomiting, diarrhea, or constipation, and interfere with the absorption and effectiveness of certain medications, including antibiotics and drugs used to treat osteoporosis, hypothyroidism, or Parkinson's disease symptoms. Always tell your doctor if you are taking an iron supplement.

16 FOOD SOURCES: ISOFLAVONES

RDA: 25 grams per day

The health benefits of isoflavones may include protection against age-related diseases such as cardiovascular disease, osteoporosis, Isoflavones are also thought to provide antioxidant activity (which is a good thing).

For many of us who have been diagnosed with thyroid disease we cannot have soy products. The good news is that there are other foods besides soy based to offer Isoflavone sources into our diets:

There are others that have a problem digesting soybeans and soy products and this causes digestive problems.

If you are **hypothyroid** most medical professionals recommend you avoid soybeans, soy sauce, soybean oil (Vegetable Oil), tofu, Edamame beans and other soy products. If soy does not bother you it is a good source of isoflavones for you and will raise your estrogen levels.

The short of it is this: If you need to raise your estrogen levels then these are good food sources to include in your diet. If you are trying to lower your estrogen then you should avoid these food sources.

Rather than alphabetical order these are in order of best source from highest to lowest:

1. Flax Seed (ground flaxseed is a great choice)
2. Soybeans and soy products (avoid with thyroid conditions)
3. Sesame Seeds and sesame seed oil
4. Chickpeas and Lentils (in moderation only)
5. Green peas
6. Garlic
7. Black Beans (in moderation only due to high carb)
8. Walnuts
9. Sunflower Seeds
10. Cucumbers
11. Squash

12. Sweet Potatoes (high carb food alert)

17 FOOD SOURCES: MAGNESIUM

According to healthline.com every cell in your body needs magnesium to function properly.

The benefits of magnesium: Magnesium can help to calm nerves and anxiety, aid in a more sound sleep, relieve constipation and it helps to regulate levels of calcium, potassium and sodium.

RDA: 400 mg for men and 320 mg daily for women
- Almonds
- Apple
- Avocado
- Broccoli
- Carrots
- Cashews
- Halibut
- Mackerel
- Pumpkin seeds
- Salmon
- Spinach (cooked/sautéed)
- Swiss Chard (cooked/sautéed)

FAQ: Which magnesium supplement should I take?
Magnesium Oxide or Magnesium Citrate?

First, always try eating a healthier diet. If you do find that you need a supplement, follow your doctors instructions. The most popular are oxide and citrate. Try one for about a month at a lower dosage say 100mg a day to simply supplement your intake from foods. If you don't find you are getting the results expected try the other. I personally take Citrate but know many people who swear by the oxide. Always consult your physician when adding supplements to your diet.

18 FOOD SOURCES: MANGANESE

AI: Approximately 2 mg per day for men and women.

Manganese is present in small amounts but it is an essential nutrient. Responsible for healthy enzyme functioning, healing from wounds, bone health and it also aids in the absorption of other nutrients your body needs. According to NaturalNews.com it also helps fight cell damaging free radicals.

Here are some of your healthiest sources to be sure you are getting the daily recommended amount of manganese.

- Leafy Green Vegetables: Cooked kale, collards, swiss chard and spinach.
- Nuts: hazelnuts, pecans, macadamia and walnuts are your best choices.
- Pineapple (the fresh ones in your produce department really are quite easy to slice and serve, ... And they taste so much better!
- Seafood (best sources: mussels, clams, crawfish, bass, trout and perch. In that order)
- Seeds
- Spices: Cloves and Saffron both are good sources.
- Tea: in particular black tea! One cup of black tea (8 oz) has approximately 1 mg (50%) of your daily recommended dosage of manganese. This means 2 cups a day is all you need.

19 FOOD SOURCES: OMEGA-3

RDA: There is no set RDA for Omega-3. Most mainstream health organizations recommend approximately 250-500mg per day for the average healthy adult.

Studies have found people with depression saw their symptoms improve after increasing their Omega-3s. Omega-3 is also known to be beneficial to your eye health, lowering triglycerides, and improve stiffness and joint pain.

Best Sources: I encourage you to search for recipes that include some of these foods. Find some favorites and make them a part of your regular diet.

- Anchovies (don't be afraid of these. Find a recipe for homemade Caesar salad dressing and give it a go! If you like Caesar Salad and its dressing you will like your homemade version. And you can freeze the leftover anchovies for the next time you make dressing.)
- Chia Seeds
- Cod Liver Oil (also an excellent source of Vit D and Vit A)
- Eggs (the whole egg)
- Flaxseed (yeah! A non-fish food source. Ground flaxseed should become your new staple in the kitchen. Its low carb and can replace flour in some recipes. I make a flourless, low carb pancake using mine. Recipe on the next page.
- Herring (kippers)
- Mackerel
- Oysters
- Salmon
- Sardines
- Spinach and Brussels Sprouts
- Walnuts

Ground Flaxseed Low Carb Pancake Recipe

- 3 tbsp. Flaxseed Meal
- Baking Soda, .25 tsp
- 1/2 teaspoon baking powder
- 1 Whole Egg
- Olive Oil, 1 tsp.
- 1 tablespoon honey
- pinch of salt

Mix well. Cook as you would any pancake but do not flip too soon. Cook over a low to medium heat. Be sure it is showing signs of browning along the edges before turning over. Flip just once for best results. Suggestions: you can, of course, add cinnamon, vanilla, and nutmeg for added flavor. Or try adding pecans! Serve with berries and Raw Honey.

(skinned, poached apricots or cooked apples and cinnamon are delicious with the Flaxseed Pancakes)

I have used this basic recipe, adding a couple tablespoons of water to thin it out and made a nice crepe with fresh fruit. Similarly you could make a cream of chicken using leftover shredded chicken and a dairy free alfredo sauce. Wrap the seasoned chicken with the very thin crepes and cover with your sauce.

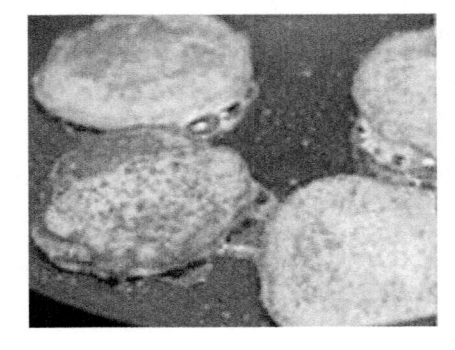

20 FOOD SOURCES: PANTOTHENIC ACID

RDA: 5 mg per day for men and women.

aka: **Vitamin B5** *which is thought to improve healing of skin wounds specifically and may play a part in lowering cholesterol. The University of Maryland Medical Center has reported that pantothenic acid, also known as B5, helps the body convert food into fuel or energy. This is one of the B vitamins which are water soluble; meaning the body does not store them.*

The umm.edu also reports a study that showed people with RA, morning stiffness and pain had lower levels of B5. Suggesting they either were not getting enough in their daily diets or that they may not be absorbing the nutrients properly.

It should be noted that taking a B Complex Supplement (which would include this vitamin) may interfere with antibiotics and with drugs used to treat Alzheimer's. Talk to your doctor about your Vitamin B consumption if you will be taking antibiotics, tetracycline, or drugs to treat Alzheimer's.

Healthy food sources:

- Avocados
- Eggs
- Liver
- Mushrooms (cooked)
- Shellfish
- Sunflower Seeds
- Sweet Potatoes

21 FOOD SOURCES: PHOSPHORUS

RDA: 700 mg per day

Phosphorus, along with calcium, work to build strong bones and teeth. Phosphorus also plays a role in ridding the body of waste in the kidneys. It eases muscle pain after a workout or labor intense day. Phosphorus, according to UMMC (University of Maryland Medical Center) is needed for the growth, maintenance and repair of all tissues and cells. Be mindful that phosphorus supplementation should always be partnered with calcium intake, whether your source is food or supplements. Phosphorus without calcium can and will pose health issues. Another reason to rely on diet sources.

Sources of Phosphorus:

- Eggs
- Garlic
- Meat
- Nuts
- Poultry
- Seafood

22 FOOD SOURCES: PHYTOESTROGENS

Also known as Estrogen. This list will be important to you if you are trying to *increase* your estrogen levels and also, these are foods you will want to avoid if you are trying to *decrease* or lower your estrogen levels.

Best Healthy Food Sources that will increase estrogen levels:

- Flaxseed: Its low carb, high fiber. I add it to smoothies but I also make my pancakes and muffins using this in place of flour.
- Sesame Seeds
- Chickpeas: Please be mindful of your portions as chickpeas are a high carb food.
- Green Peas

When you are trying to raise your levels, like that of estrogen, in the body, it happens as it compounds in the body. In other words, you need to incorporate food sources on a regular, ongoing basis. Alternatively, if you are trying to rid your body or lower your levels, because it may have compounded in the body, it may take up to a month of elimination before being able to notice a significant change in how you feel.

23 FOOD SOURCES: POTASSIUM

RDA: Because lack of potassium is rare, there is no RDA for this mineral. However, it is thought that *1600 to 2000 mg daily is adequate*. If you do take a potassium supplement be sure you are also considering how much potassium you are getting in the foods you eat.

Potassium maintains fluid volume inside and outside of cells and prevents the excess rise of blood pressure with increased sodium intake.

Foods with higher amounts of Potassium:

- Apricots (skinned, poached apricots are delicious with the Flaxseed Pancakes)
- Artichokes
- Avocados
- Bananas (high sugar warning)
- Beets
- Brussels sprouts
- Cantaloupe
- Oranges
- Parsnips
- Potatoes (nightshade warning)
- Prunes
- Pumpkin
- Spinach
- Sweet Potatoes (high carbohydrate alert)
- Swiss Chard (green leafy)
- Tomatoes (nightshade warning)
- Zucchini

There are some of you, due to health issues, that need to eat a LOW potassium diet. You should avoid the list of foods above. I wanted to include healthy options that have less than 100 mg of potassium per half cup for those of you who are trying to keep your potassium intake down but are looking for healthy food choices

- Blueberries
- Cabbage
- Cranberries
- Cucumber
- Endive
- Okra
- Onion
- Green Peas
- Pineapple
- Raspberries
- Watermelon

24 FOOD SOURCES: PROTEIN

We are all aware that meat is one of our best sources of protein, but there are other options and not just high carb legumes!

RDA for women: 46 grams each day and 56 grams for men per some sources.

Proteins:
Ten to 35 percent of calories should come from lean protein.
Protein is the major structural component of cells and is responsible for the building and repair of body tissues. Protein is broken down into amino acids, which are building blocks of protein. Nine of the 20 amino acids, known as essential amino acids, must be provided in the diet as they cannot be synthesized in the body. Ten to 35 percent of your daily calories should come from lean protein sources such as low carb vegetables, low-fat meat, seafood, or eggs.

Others, like The Institute of Medicine, which I recommend, suggest your RDA of protein should be determined by your weight. **To** determine how much protein you should be eating, multiply your weight by .4 grams. For example if you weigh 140 pounds, you need about 56 grams of protein per day.   140 x .4 = 56

- Almonds
- Artichokes
- Asparagus
- Avocado
- Beef
- Broccoli
- Brussels Sprouts
- Chicken
- Eggs
- Kale and Spinach
- Mushrooms
- Oats (grain alert for those avoiding grains)
- Peas, green
- Pumpkin Seeds

- Seafood – especially tuna

Your body turns the protein you get from your diet into amino acids, which are responsible for continuously replacing proteins in your body, according to the Centers for Disease Control and Prevention. This process is essential for survival and for your cells, tissues and muscles to work properly.

Proteins make up your bones, muscles, and skin. in fact, proteins are in every living cell in your body. your cells and proteins perform many functions, including:

- helping to break down food for energy
- building structures
- breaking down toxins

25 FOOD SOURCES: SELENIUM

RDA: 55 mcg per day for men and women.

Selenium helps keep your thyroid functioning properly. Selenium, which is nutritionally essential for humans, plays a critical role in reproduction, thyroid hormone metabolism, DNA synthesis, and protection from oxidative damage and infection.

Excellent sources of Selenium:

- Asparagus
- Beef liver
- Broccoli
- Brazil Nuts
- Carrots
- Eggs
- Grass fed beef
- Green peas
- Halibut
- Kale (cooked)
- Mushrooms (cooked)
- Onions
- Oysters
- Poultry
- Sunflower seeds
- Pork
- Salmon
- Sardines
- Spinach
- Yellowfin tuna

26 FOOD SOURCES: SODIUM

RDA: The American Heart Association recommends you limit your sodium intake to 1,500 milligrams or less per day.

How much sodium is in table salt?
- 1/4 teaspoon salt = 575 mg sodium
- 1/2 teaspoon salt = 1,150 mg sodium
- 3/4 teaspoon salt = 1,725 mg sodium
- 1 teaspoon salt = 2,300 mg sodium

Sodium helps to maintain fluid volume outside of the cells and helps cells to function normally. Keep intake under 1500 milligrams per day.

Sodium also occurs naturally in unprocessed foods. This fact is often overlooked. All the more reason to cut back on table salt and begin to omit processed and pre-prepared foods that have added sodium.

Suggestion: Start to look at the label and sodium content of everything you consume. Everything.

Sodium is known to cause blood pressure to rise but even if you do not have high blood pressure, excess sodium is also known to be one of the complex root causes of stroke. The medical industry will tell you that high blood pressure is first and foremost inherited from family. That is not a free pass to make it worse by eating foods that cause it to be more threatening to your own health. Instead, it should cause you take pause in your dietary choices. Do everything you can to offset this gene. It really can make a difference!

Suggestion: While most of your vegetables and fruits should come in fresh or frozen form, we do occasionally buy canned fruits and vegetables. Be sure when choosing canned foods that you choose NO SALT varieties when available. I find they actually taste more like fresh! Never rely on the front of the label verbiage. Such as, "reduced salt" "reduced sodium". Always, always, always check out the label. If it has a label you should feel obliged to read it. Take note of the ingredients list and the Nutritional Values stated.

Case and Point: I purchased a product labeled Organic Chicken Broth and when I got home I turned it around to read the label. The ingredients list did not have chicken broth or stock listed at all. On another occasion I purchased dried blueberries for a recipe. When I got home and looked at the back of the packaged of what was called "Dried Blueberries" on the front realized that it was dried grapes infused with blueberry juice. That is not the same thing.

READ YOUR LABELS.

Be sure that you are considering all the sodium you are taking in from all sources when trying to limit sodium to less than 1500 mg per day.

Foods with the highest amounts of sodium and a good reason to cut these foods should not be a part of your daily diet:

- Bread (sodium quoted is generally per slice)
- Cured Meat like bacon and sausage, and....
- Lunchmeat
- Packaged Processed foods

Beverages with naturally occurring sodium:

- Beer: 240 Grams per cup
- Coffee 230 Grams per cup
- Cola 240 Grams per cup
- Red and White Wine 100 Grams per cup

While all vegetables are naturally low in sodium, many *DO* contain sodium and should be considered when tallying up your daily sodium consumption.

The following are considered naturally SODIUM FREE FOODS!

- **Apple 2 mg per medium apple**
- **Apricot**
- **Asparagus**
- **Avocado**
- **Green Beans**
- **Blackberries**
- **Blueberries**
- **Cucumber**
- **Endive**
- **Garlic**
- **Lettuce**
- **Limes**
- **Oranges**
- **Peaches**
- **Pears**
- **Raspberries**
- **Strawberries**
- **Yellow Squash**

Low Sodium Unprocessed Foods:

- Broccoli 49 mg per cup
- Brussels Sprouts
- Cabbage
- Cantaloupe
- Carrots
- Cauliflower
- Celery
- Chickpeas
- Collard Greens (leafy green)
- Grapes
- Lentils
- Honeydew Melon
- Mushrooms
- Okra
- Onions
- Parsley
- Radishes
- Rhubarb
- Spaghetti Squash
- Sweet Potatoes

27 FOOD SOURCES: VITAMIN A

RDA: 900 mcg daily which is the equivalent of 3000 IU

We need vitamin A for healthy skin and mucus membranes, our immune system, good eye health and vision.

Because Vitamin A is a fat soluble nutrient it needs to be consumed with fat for proper absorption. Be sure to choose healthy fats!

Best sources of Vitamin A:

- Butter: Real Butter; choose unsalted
- Egg (the whole egg: it's in the yolk!)
- Liver

Many people who do not easily digest dairy can in fact process real butter. Others cannot. This is something you will have to find out for yourself in your own unique situations. Consult a doctor if you feel uncertain.

Why aren't carrots listed? Carrots actually have beta carotene. In most healthy adults beta carotene is converted, by the body, into Vitamin A so it isn't that including carrots is exactly incorrect. However, I wanted to only include true Vitamin A enriched foods for everyone so as not to mislead those with thyroid and other disorders that may inhibit that conversion.

28 FOOD SOURCES: VITAMIN B1(THIAMIN)

RDA: 1-2 mg per day. Such a low amount indicates your best source would be through your food intake. If your doctor has instructed you to take a supplement follow your physicians advice as to per day amounts for your condition.

You will notice that in the supplement isle at the store, Vitamin B1 Thiamin comes in amounts as much as 250 mg per tablet. That is for persons who are severely deficient and have been instructed by their doctor to take the upper level dosage and not the average person.

Vitamin B1, an essential nutrient, maintains cellular function and various organ function in the body. A person can find themselves deficient for a variety of reasons: poor diet, illness, poor absorption.

Chemicals in coffee and tea called tannins can react with thiamine, converting it to a form that is difficult for the body to take in. This could lead to thiamine deficiency

Seafood

Raw freshwater fish and shellfish contain chemicals that destroy thiamine. Eating a lot of raw fish or shellfish can contribute to thiamine deficiency. However, cooked fish and seafood are OK.

People take thiamine supplements for conditions related to low levels of thiamine (thiamine deficiency syndromes), including beriberi and inflammation of the nerves (neuritis) associated with pellagra or pregnancy.

Thiamine is also used for digestive problems including poor appetite, ulcerative colitis, and ongoing diarrhea.

Reasons to eat foods with Thiamine:

Thiamine can boost the immune system, ease diabetic pain, heart disease, alcoholism, aging, canker sores, vision problems such as cataracts and glaucoma, and motion sickness.
Some people find thiamine helps in maintaining a positive mental attitude; enhancing learning abilities; increasing energy; fighting stress; and preventing memory loss, including Alzheimer's disease.

Here are foods you can incorporate into your daily diet to increase the Vitamin B1 in your system. Deficiencies can lead to fatigue and gastrointestinal problems.

- Asparagus
- Acorn, Butternut and Hubbard Squash
- Brussels sprouts
- Cabbage
- Cauliflower
- Cumin
- Flaxseed
- Green beans
- Green Peas
- Kale
- Nuts: particularly brazil nuts, macadamia, pecans and cashews.
- Oats (grain)
- Parsley
- Pork
- Romaine lettuce (have you tried it grilled yet?)
- Seafood like salmon, trout, tuna and mackerel.
- Spinach
- Sunflower seeds
- Sweet potato
- Swiss chard
- Tuna
- Watermelon

29 FOOD SOURCES: VITAMIN B12

RDA: 2.4 mcg per day for the average healthy person.

Vitamin B12 allows for healthy red blood cell formation and neurological function. Proper absorption is as important as getting it into your regular diet.

Best natural food sources for Vitamin B12:

- Clams: cooked
- Beef Liver

I want to stop here and point out that clams and beef liver are far and above your best sources but if you are vegetarian or do not care for either of those; the following foods are also good food sources!

- Beef top sirloin
- Chicken
- Eggs
- Haddock
- Salmon
- Trout
- Tuna
- Shitake Mushrooms (Cooked)
- Soybeans, Soy sauce and other soy products (*to be avoided if you are hypothyroid*) *It should also be noted that the digestive system has a very difficult time breaking down soy products and so it is suggested by some professionals to avoid soy products if you live with digestive issues. Speak to your doctor or try an elimination diet to find out your tolerance level.*

30 FOOD SOURCES: VITAMIN B2(RIBOFLAVIN)

RDA: In adults, the average daily **riboflavin** intake from foods is 2.5 mg in men and 1.8 mg in women

Vitamin B2, also known as Riboflavin, is essential for energy metabolism and cellular processes in the body.

- Almonds, Pine Nuts, and cashews
- Asparagus
- Beef steak (lean)
- Collard Greens
- Eggs:
- Mackerel, salmon, trout and tuna
- **Mushrooms:** (white, portabella, cremini) [cooked]
- Pork (lean pork like pork sirloin chops, ground pork (not breakfast sausage), pork shoulder and pork loin are best choices.
- Sesame seeds
- Seafood like oysters, clams and mussels
- Spinach, Beet greens

31 FOOD SOURCES: VITAMIN B3(NIACIN)

RDA: 14 milligrams each day for women. 16 milligrams for men.

Niacin is known to be beneficial to lowering cholesterol, boosting brain function, healthy skin, and may help with joint mobility

Cited study: ncbi.nlm.nih.gov/pubmed/8841834

Best food sources for Niacin:

- Asparagus
- Beef
- Beets
- Chicken
- green peas
- Halibut
- Mushrooms
- Peanuts
- Salmon
- Sunflower Seeds
- Tuna
- Turkey

According to lpi.oregonstate.edu/mic/vitamins/niacin
the recommended daily consumption of niacin is 16 mg for men and 14 mg for women. If you are eating a variety of the vitamin B3 rich foods listed above you probably don't need a supplement. Absorption is key. So if you feel you are eating the right foods but still are falling short of this or any other vitamin or nutrient be sure to read over the chapter on absorption, Chapter 58.

32 FOOD SOURCES: VITAMIN B6

RDA: 1.5 mg for women and approximately 2 mg per day for men.

MayoClinic.org reports that Vitamin B6, also known as pyridoxine, is necessary in the bodies process of making serotonin. Serotonin is a chemical that transmits signals to the brain. Vitamin B6 also supports forming healthy nerve cells. They also state that mild deficiency is common and can cause some health issues for some people.

Food sources to include in your diet:

- Carrots
- Eggs (the whole egg including the yolk)
- Green Peas
- Liver
- Seafood
- Spinach

33 FOOD SOURCES: VITAMIN C

RDA: 60-90 mg per day for both men and women.

*Vitamin C, also listed in ingredients as **ascorbic acid** is one of the most effective and safest* **nutrients**. *It is an antioxidant necessary for the synthesis of collagen, which provides structure to blood vessels, helps muscles, bones and ligaments stay strong.*

Best sources for Vitamin C:

- Artichokes
- Asparagus
- Broccoli
- Cabbage
- Cauliflower (when cooked)
- Citrus fruits like oranges (fresh fruit Not orange juice)
- Brussels Sprouts
- Cucumber
- Green leafy vegetables: Like Kale and Spinach
- Green Beans
- Okra
- Onions
- Radishes
- Summer Squash

Also a good list to reference for those who want their quota of Vitamin C but are avoiding citrus.

If you are avoiding citrus but have a dish that calls for lemon juice or lime juice you can use the zest of a lime, lemon or orange. The zest does not contain the active ingredients that the juice contains.

34 FOOD SOURCES: VITAMIN D

My first suggestion to anyone striving to get more Vitamin D is to go outdoors every day for at least 15 minutes. You must spend that time in an area outdoors that the sky is not blocked by an overhang, inside of a vehicle or other apparatus like an umbrella. Spending time outdoors daily in natural light has other benefits for your mood and sleep cycles and not just on your absorption of Vitamin D. Strive for a minimum of 15 consecutive minutes a day. My second is to include the foods listed below that are excellent sources.

RDA: Recommended Daily Intake is 400-600 IU of vitamin D per day (5 mcg)

Consult with your doctor if you are unsure as some health issues may affect your vitamin D levels.

Vitamin D helps to regulate the absorption of calcium as well as phosphorus. It is also thought to enhance the function of the immune system. Vitamin D can play a big part in healthy bones and teeth while improving your resistance against some diseases.

Food Sources

- Cod Liver Oil (not a fan? Here are some other foods J)
- Egg Yolks (whole egg)
- Herring and Sardines
- Mushrooms: wild more so than commercially grown. Also, all mushrooms are more nutritious when eaten cooked, rather than raw. Even a quick sauté will do!
- Oysters
- Shrimp
- Wild Salmon

Not a seafood fan? Try committing to 3 times a week to get your palate adjusted. I started with Cod. It's a nice subtle mild white fish.

In a 2006 study published in the Journal of the American Medical Association (jama.com) Vitamin D can reduce risk of multiple sclerosis.

Likewise, a 2008 study found Vitamin D can reduce your risk of heart disease and a 2010 study showed Vitamin D reduces the chance of getting the flu.

Some research has indicated that Vitamin D may play a role in warding off depression and anxiety as well as symptoms of those thought to have fibromyalgia.

Getting outside and making good food choices are great but you should also be sure to not hinder Vitamin D getting into your system. These things can hinder your ability to maintain adequate amounts of Vitamin D:

- Living in an area with high pollution
- Using sunscreen (use only when spending more than 15 minutes outdoors)
- Spending time indoors
- Living in big cities where buildings block the sun

A word of caution to those of you with darker skin. Having darker skin, i.e.: higher levels of melanin, the less Vitamin D the skin can absorb. Be sure to have your Vitamin D checked annually and follow a diet and lifestyle to maintain adequate levels of Vitamin D.

Symptoms of Vitamin D deficiency in adults can include:

- Unexplained tiredness, aches, pains and a general feeling of unwellness
- Bone and muscle pain or weakness
- Feeling fatigue in the legs after going up or down a flight of stairs
- Feeling fatigue in the arms after using your arms for a period of time.

Talk to your physician if you are experiencing these symptoms without any other obvious explanation like the flu.

35 FOOD SOURCES: VITAMIN E

Vitamin E is common in many food sources. Great news as it is essential for the body to function normally. Vitamin E is first and foremost an antioxidant. It is also known to assist in the protection of LDL cholesterol, also known as the "bad" cholesterol. Vitamin E plays a role in red blood cell formation and helps the body use Vitamin K.

RDA: The average healthy person only needs approximately 15mg per day of Vitamin E and yet research shows most people fall short. Easy enough to get from the foods you eat and not need to take a supplement. Your two best sources are dark green leafy vegetables and Sunflower Seeds and Sunflower oil.

Here are some of the highest food sources for Vitamin E

- Almonds
- Atlantic Salmon
- Asparagus
- Avocado
- Blackberries
- Brazil Nuts (also a good source of selenium)
- Broccoli
- Carrots
- Cod
- Dark green leafy vegetables **(Best Source!)**
- Green beans
- Kiwi
- Olives (black olives are green olives that have been left on the tree)
- Olive Oil
- Rainbow Trout
- Red peppers (nightshade warning)
- Shrimp and Sardines
- Sunflower Seeds and Sunflower Oil (*Best Source!*)
- Swiss Chard and Spinach (dark green leafy)
- Turnip greens (dark green leafy)
- Wheat Germ (gluten alert)

36 FOOD SOURCES: VITAMIN K

Vitamin K is required for proper blood clotting.

RDA: women 90 mcg daily ~ 120 mcg men

The following foods have higher amounts of Vitamin K:

- Asparagus
- Broccoli
- Brussel Sprouts
- Cabbage
- Cauliflower
- Cucumbers
- Dried Fruits (high sugar alert)
- Green Leafy vegetables like kale, spinach and collards
- Lettuce: all varieties
- Many herbs are high in Vitamin K like basil, sage, thyme, parsley, cilantro and chives.
- Okra
- Olive Oil

If you take a blood thinner like warfarin (Coumadin) your doctor has probably talked to you about being mindful of how much Vitamin K you consume. Talk to your doctor about keeping your diet consistent as far as foods that contain Vitamin K so that your dosage of warfarin does not constantly need adjusted. For example, if you eat a salad everyday make sure you eat it every single day and in the same portion. Changing your intake of a food that is known to have Vitamin K like leafy greens can cause your dosage to be adjusted.

If you do take Coumadin (warfarin), it's important to have about the same amount of Vitamin K-containing foods every day. Too much vitamin K in your diet may lessen the effectiveness of Coumadin.

While the foods listed above thicken the blood, helping your body to form healthy blood clots as needed when you have a cut, the foods below are reported to aide in thinning the blood:

They include:

- berries, grapes, grapefruits, pineapple, and pomegranates
- dark chocolate
- fish like mackerel, trout, herring, albacore tuna, and salmon
- garlic
- green tea
- onions
- tree nuts like walnuts, almonds, hazelnuts, cashews, pistachios, and brazil nuts

37 FOOD SOURCES: ZINC

RDA: Overall, resources state the daily requirement for Zinc is 8 mg for adult women and 11 mg for adult men

zinc plays an important role in the release of certain hormones.

Oysters contain more zinc per serving than any other food, but red meat and poultry provide the majority of zinc in the American diet. Other good food sources include beans, nuts, certain types of seafood (such as crab and lobster)

- broccoli
- cashews
- chia seeds
- Chick peas, lentils, black beans (high carb alert)
- garlic
- kale
- meat
- mushrooms
- Oysters
- pecans
- Poultry
- Red
- spinach

38 WATER

According to the University of Missouri; Water is the single most important nutrient of life. Without water, no metabolic and physiological processes within the body can occur.

Water is necessary for the movement of nutrients to the cells, removal of waste products from these cells, mineral or acid base balance, protection of nervous system, lubrication of joints, flushes bacteria from the bladder, aides digestion, maintains sodium balance, and body temperature control.

Other signs of water being essential are that water is required in amounts larger than any other nutrient and represents approximately 50 to 80 % of body weight depending on age and fat content of the individual.

The health and medical community has stated a person needs 1.5 to 2 liters of water each day to replace what is lost through urinating, sweating, breathing, tears and watery eyes, poor diets, medications, and stress. Not replacing water loss is what leads to dehydration.

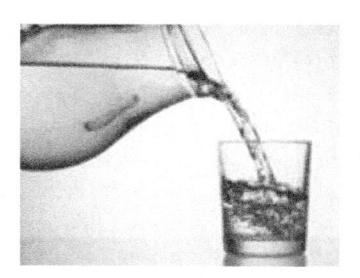

Types of Water:
Distilled Water: Distilled water, also known as demineralized water is a most pure water. All of the minerals and salt have been removed by the process of reverse osmosis and distillation. It is an absolute pure for of water. A small portion of the population has chosen distilled water as their water of choice. If you do drink distilled water as a matter of choice, be sure you are otherwise eating a very healthy diet that gives you the minerals you need that are not present in distilled water like potassium, chloride and magnesium. I personally drink distilled water only due to a process of elimination. All other waters caused stomach upset and digestive issues. Having said that, my diet is 99% unprocessed, fresh, healthy foods along with a few supplements.
Mineral Water: Mineral water naturally contains minerals. Mineral water comes from underground sources which results in the natural minerals in the water like calcium, magnesium and manganese. True Mineral Water cannot have further minerals added and cannot be subjected to treatment before packing for public consumption.
Purified Water: Purified water has been purified in a treatment plant. Purifying water means all bacteria and contaminants have been removed. Purified water can be purchased or can also be obtained by adding a water purifier to your faucet.
Sparkling Water: Water that has been carbonated. When purchasing it is good to read the label to find out what type of water was originally used to carbonate if you are particular about the variety of water you drink.
Spring Water: Spring water is the result of rain that does not end up deep in the ground and instead leaks to the surface as a spring or through the crevice of a rock.
Tap Water: Come from the tap. Considered safe to drink by way of city, state and municipal regulations. It is highly recommended to pay attention to the annual letters from your water company about the contents and possible warnings in your tap water. Tap water in the United States has been fluoridated. In other words fluoride has been added to the water in an effort to reduce tooth decay. If you do not drink tap water be sure you are using a fluoride rinse to protect your teeth from decay and cavities. Having said that, we are becoming more and more aware that some people have a sensitivity or allergy to fluoride or feel fluoride is to blame for some of our health issues. Fluoride has been banned in some countries citing it's toxic nature to humans. Consult with your doctor and/or dentist for the care of your teeth and possible water choices.
Well Water: Rain seeps into the ground, into the soil and into underground lakes. It is important to test the safety of your well water on a regular basis.

The recommended 1.5 to 3 liters (4.25-12 cups a day) of water equates to:

- 1 liter equals about 4 cups (there are 8 ounces in one cup)
- (8) 8-ounce glasses per day. 64 ounces (8x8) is equal to about 2 liters, or half a gallon.

If you are tired of counting and tracking your daily water intake here are some simple habits to form.

Personally I find that, with the proper healthy diet, one needs to follow just a few basic rules to stay hydrated and get plenty of water for the body to function properly.

1. Choose water as your choice of beverage with your meals. Every meal.
2. Always start your day with a 10 ounce glass of room temperature water consumed over the course of about 30 minutes. Consider that you have not had any water for at least 8-10 hours upon waking. The first thing you put in your body, and directly in your stomach should be plain water; not coffee, tea, juice or cola. Wait to have your coffee or tea, if you drink it, until after your glass of water.
3. Always take medications, supplements, over-the-counter meds, and vitamins with at least a 10 ounce glass of plain water unless otherwise instructed by your physician or the pharmacist. The exception would be at bed time only.
4. Drink at least 10 ounces of water *prior* to any workout or physical activity. And of course during and after as needed.
5. Eat foods that have a high water content as a part of your regular diet.

3 ten ounce glasses (one with each meal) = 30 ounces
1 ten ounce upon rising in the morning = 10 ounces
1 ten ounce glass before exercise/activity = 10 ounces
1 ten ounce glass with medications = 10 ounces

This, regimen can easily add up to approximately 64 ounces per day. Any shortage will most likely be made up with:

1. hydrating foods as a part of your daily diet (Very Important!)
2. Broth and broth based soups
3. unsweetened tea
4. unsweetened coffee

Eat Your Water

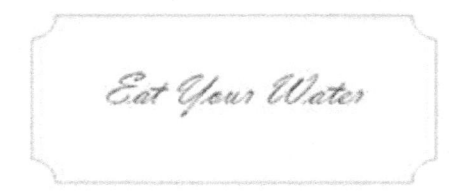

There was a time when we purposely avoided foods that were "mostly water" but no more!

Foods high in water content are a great way to stay hydrated as most of them are also low carb, fresh, unprocessed and full of nutrients.

The following foods are in order from the foods with the *highest water content first*. All are not only excellent sources of hydrating foods but contain much needed nutrients that will be better absorbed due to the foods water content!

1. Cucumbers
2. Iceberg Lettuce (try eating a wedge after a workout or after you get home from work each day)
3. Celery
4. Radishes
5. Tomatoes (nightshade alert!)
6. Green Bell peppers (nightshade alert)
7. Cauliflower
8. Watermelon
9. Spinach
10. Strawberries
11. Broccoli
12. Grapefruit (be careful of medication interactions and also a citrus food alert)
13. Carrots
14. Cantaloupe

Look for fresh recipes using these ingredients. Eat simply by merely washing and slicing or do a simple preparation of slicing and tossing with one another with a bit of oil, salt and pepper. Have you tried a nightshade free watermelon salsa?

Hydrating Cucumber Vegetable Dip Recipe

This is a very hydrating and fresh dip that can also be used on sandwiches in place of mayo. This is Very low carb, dairy free, gluten free, nightshade free, soy free and grain free. It is also all fresh and very healthy.

- 1 peeled cucumber, chopped
- ½ cup chopped iceberg lettuce
- 4 tablespoons Sunflower Oil
- 4 tablespoons water
- A pinch of salt and a pinch of black pepper
- 1 capful of Raw, Unfiltered Apple Cider Vinegar

Optional additions to the blender for a different flavor and texture profile:

- 1/8 cup chopped parsley or cilantro
- One drained can of artichokes

Place oil, vinegar, and water in your chopper or blender first. Then add the remaining ingredients. Blend to the consistency you like. Some prefer a more rustic chunky dip while sometimes, like if making a sandwich spread, you may prefer a smoother dip. If you find it is too thin add more lettuce.

Once removed and placed in a bowl, adjust seasonings and vinegar/oil as needed and stir well.

The addition of other seasonings is optional. It is recommended that these seasonings be added after removing from the blender as sometimes it can turn them bitter.

Some suggestions:

- Italian Seasoning
- Onion Powder
- Garlic Powder

39 UNDERSTANDING HOW FOODS DIGEST

For the average healthy person this may not be of much significance, however, for those with digestive problems this is a big deal to understand how foods digest in the system.

Water actually take 20-30 minutes to digest. This is why you can feel full for about half hour after drinking a glass of water. It is also why those of you who have a problem with gerd can sometimes simply take a drink of water and feel discomfort.

- Fruit and broth based soups with cooked vegetables take about 45 minutes to digest through the digestive tract.
- Vegetables (cooked) take approximately 45 minutes
- Legumes, grains and starches like bread, pasta and potatoes take up to 3 hours to digest completely and move thru the digestive tract.
- Meat, Fish, Poultry and eggs take the longest: 4-8 hours.

Logic may tell you that you should eat meat first since it takes longer to digest when, in fact, it is the opposite.

Imagine a tube, like your digestive tract.
If you eat meat for breakfast, or early in the day, even lunchtime, anything you eat within the next four(4) to eight(8) hours will be stuck behind the meat because it has not had time to digest and move through the digestive tract.

This can cause constipation, gerd, abdominal pain and discomfort.

For this reason, those who experience digestive issues may find relief in eating their foods in a mindful manner.

1. Fruit for breakfast if you eat fruit at all. Fruit has plenty of time to digest and move on before you have lunch in 3 or 4 hours. If you are trying to lose weight, doing an elimination period or cleansing your palate do not eat fruit at all during the first 45-60 days. You will find other breakfast options later in the book and in the *Companion Workbook.

2. Vegetables for lunch and perhaps broth if in a soup. Again, this will have time to digest before supper.

3. Protein for supper: If you eat meat, save it for your evening meal so that it has overnight to digest before you have breakfast in the morning.

The Digestive System

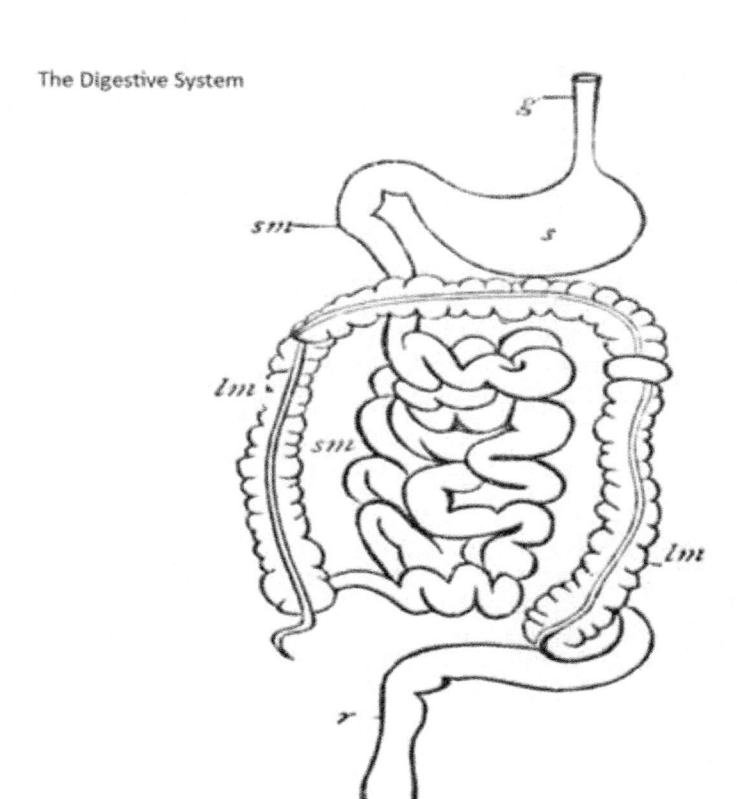

For those living with gerd, digestive issues and constipation:

1. Fruit digest the quickest. Eat it for breakfast so it doesn't get stuck behind meat that can take up to 6 hours to digest. This can cause constipation, cramping and digestive problems for some. **2. Eat vegetables** for lunch. The fruit should have had time to digest and clear the way! Vegetables take a few hours to digest. **3. Save meat** for your evening meal as meat can take up to 6 hours to digest. Eaten earlier it can cause a back-up. Blocking other foods from being digested in the timeframe they were meant to.

40 BROTH AND STOCK

Broth can be an extremely healthy and healing food! But only if it is a pure broth. Broth (or stock) is also low carb; so healthy waistline friendly.

If you are eating dairy free broth is also an excellent replacement for milk when making sauces, gravies and creamy soups.

Homemade chicken stock delivers 3.8 milligrams of niacin per cup. Niacin is a B vitamin that helps you metabolize the foods you eat, and it also promotes the normal function of your nerves, skin and digestive system, the University of Maryland Medical Center notes. Those 3.8 milligrams translate to 27 percent of the 14 milligrams women need each day and 24 percent of the 16 milligrams men should have daily. Homemade chicken broth/stock also provides small amounts of potassium, iron and zinc, as well.

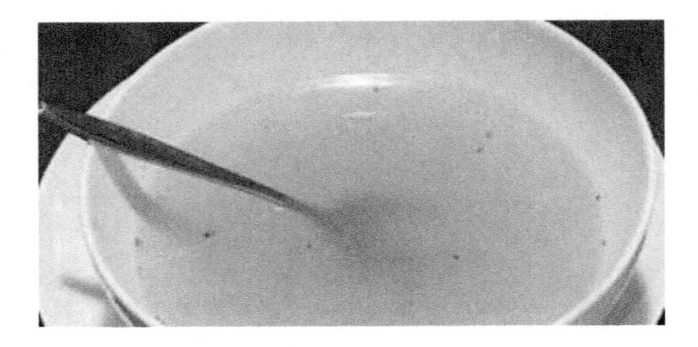

What is the difference in broth and stock?

Broth is made by boiling meat or vegetables in water.

Stock is made by boiling bones in water.

Nevertheless, stock contains collagen, marrow, amino acids and minerals. These may protect the digestive tract, improve sleep and support joint health.

Parsley, oregano and thyme, for example, are all sources of antioxidants that are commonly used in broth. And certain cooking methods, including simmering, actually increase their antioxidant capacity.

Onions and garlic also have their own unique benefits, including antibacterial, anti-inflammatory and immune-boosting properties.

I like to get the best of both worlds by making my own stock/broth using bone-in meats like bone-in chicken thighs, poaching chicken breast with the rib, bone-in roast and bone-in beef shanks.

Poaching is a great technique to create both/stock to be used during that same meal or next day.

Poach: cook by simmering in a small amount of liquid. Water, broth/stock, or even non-dairy milk.

Poaching chicken breasts is a simple and delicious way to enjoy poultry.
Rub your chicken breast "with the rib" (bone-in), with oil, salt and pepper. Brown on both sides in a hot skillet turning only once. Wait until the first side is a nice golden brown before turning over. Even if you are using skinless breasts. (this can also be done with bone-in chicken thighs of course). Once both sides are browned remove temporarily from the skillet. Add just a small amount of water and scrape the bottom of the skillet to loosen up any renderings. Return the chicken to the skillet and add more water until the chicken is halfway covered. The top of the chicken should not be covered in water. Bring to a simmer and cover with a lid. Set your timer for 10-20 minutes depending on the size of your chicken pieces. Try this simple method first to see how you like the basic poached chicken. Then, the next time remember you can always add different seasonings for a different taste profile. Some suggestions would be to add cumin when adding the salt and pepper, or perhaps Italian seasoning. You could also add garlic and/or onions to the water while simmering.

The broth created from the poaching can be saved for another meal, or you can use it to make gravy by thickening it with a roux slurry. No milk needed!

Or, use it to make mashed cauliflower. Put cooled, cooked cauliflower in the blender and part of your broth, a little at a time, and blend. You want the mashed cauliflower the consistency of mashed potatoes so not too much broth. I like to put a can of drained canned asparagus in the blender with just a bit of the broth, add salt and pepper to taste. Remove and add to the skillet after removing the cooked chicken. Add garlic and perhaps a smidgeon of parmesan cheese, a capful of apple cider vinegar or a teaspoon of mustard. The parm, vinegar or mustard will give it a bright note! Sage is also a good seasoning to add if using the mustard. This makes a nice asparagus sauce for the chicken you just made. It's also low carb, gluten free, and dairy free if you choose the mustard or vinegar instead of the parmesan cheese.

The crock pot is a great source for making more than you would need in one meal so you can put some in the freezer.

Make your homemade broth the way you like it. I like mine to be a pure broth. Meaning I do not add all the vegetables and herbs I've seen in other methods. I will sometimes add a few garlic cloves but nothing else.

I freeze my broth two ways. I put part of it in freezer containers for when I want to make soup or need larger amounts. But I also freeze some in ice cube trays and once frozen transfer the cubes into freezer bags. Then, on the occasion I just need a small amount of broth I can simply grab a couple of the frozen cubes.

41 FOOD FOR WHAT AILS YOU

Some foods help while others hinder. It won't do you much good to eat turmeric daily for inflammation while consuming a diet that is highly inflammatory.

Same goes with any prescriptions or supplements you take.

Whatever you may be doing to help yourself you should also pay attention to not consume foods that will hinder their ability to help you. If strong scents cause you a headache you generally not only take an over the counter medication for the headache but you try to avoid being around strong scents.

Same goes with inflammation and digestive issues.

In the following chapters we will touch on the connection between foods and health issues and conditions that may be avoided completely or at minimum lessen the symptoms you are experiencing.

42 FOODS THAT ARE KNOWN TO CAUSE INFLAMMATION

- Sugar
- Dairy
- Nightshades
- Gluten
- Grains
- Overly processed foods
- Tobacco (a nightshade)

I encourage you to cleanse your Palate of these foods. Keeping inflammation at bay is your number one reason. You should also know that years of eating these foods dulls the palate and, for many, it is why they do not like vegetables, or why you do not crave healthy foods.

These processed foods causes faux hunger pangs and dulls your taste buds to the point you cannot taste the true flavor of unprocessed healthy foods any longer.

This can be corrected with a palate cleanse. You goal is to go at least 60 days consecutive without any processed foods, sugars, dairy, nightshades, glutens, grains, or legumes. Most people find they have a problem cheating and it takes, on average, a year to finally be able to 60 straight days without cheating.

Start your countdown on a wall calendar so you can see it at a glance. Day one you will write 60. Day 2 you will write 59, and so on. Counting down the days.

Write down on a wall calendar when you cheat. Then, the following day on the calendar start your countdown over: 60, 59, 58.....

In the next few pages you will find an explanation of each of the six groups that cause inflammation listed above.

Inflammation is associated with:

Asthma
Allergies
Arthritis: Rheumatoid and Psoriatic
Athlete's foot
Celiac
Congestion
Crohns disease
Cysts
Fibromyalgia
Headaches; frequent
Hives
IBS
Joint Pain
Lupus
Migraines
Psoriasis
Stiffness
Thyroid disease
Vitiligo

.....and that is a short list. We could all benefit from eating a diet and living a lifestyle that keeps inflammation at low, healthy levels. Exercise is a great anti-inflammatory as is the unprocessed foods low carb no sugar diet discussed in this book.

43 SUGAR

The first thing you should know about sugar, even sugars from healthy sources, is that sugar is a carbohydrate. Four (4) grams of sugar contains 16 calories. Four grams is equal to one teaspoon.

If you are diabetic follow your physicians instructions and the GI.

If you are still eating packaged foods with an ingredient list it can be very helpful to know the many other names sugar can show up as:

Caramel
Fructose
Sweetener
Corn syrup
Dextrose
Glucose
Lactose
Maltodextrin
Maltose
Sucrose
Xylitol

"Sugar Free" generally means artificially sweetened. Whereas Unsweetened means no sweetener has been added. Another reason to get away from eating packaged foods! You don't have to read and understand all the labels.

Foods that have natural sugars are fruits, gluten and dairy products.

Foods with naturally occurring sugars like that from fresh fruit and raw honey does have its benefits but one must still be mindful of your portions as this can cause weight gain and problems if you are diabetic or undiagnosed borderline diabetic. These foods can also cause inflammation. Unlike non-starchy vegetables where you need not worry so much about portion control.

Fresh fruits like bananas, apples, grapes and pears have approximately 20 carbs per serving. Dried fruits have a much higher carb count as the sugar gets concentrated in the process of the fruit being dehydrated.

Too much sugar, of any kind, causes inflammation. Besides arthritis, inflammation can cause acne, migraines, allergies, gut problems, stiffness even without arthritis, and more.

If you have a sweet tooth you may find this hard to believe but you can, in fact, adapt and live without sweets. Sweets are not necessary to the diet. Sweets and desserts are addictive to the brain and much like nicotine, it is consuming it that brings on the next craving. So the best way to combat cravings is to stop it all together. 100%. I have found most people who will eliminate all sugar for at least 3 months without cheating find they no longer have the cravings. I do have a piece of cheesecake once a year on my birthday but I must say that I do not enjoy it as much as I once did. Eliminating sugar brings your palate back to life and vegetables I once thought were bland taste full of flavor and those are the foods I now crave. This can happen for you too!

Don't allow yourself to get caught up in eating natural sweeteners. Even natural sugars from fruit and honey is bad for you if not kept in check. This is one of the few times I agree that moderation and portion control needs to become a discipline and that is with natural sources of sugar such as fruit and honey. Any other sources like white and brown sugar should either be banned completely or put on the ONLY THE SMALLEST OF SMALL PORTIONS just several TIMES A YEAR list.

Any time you eat sugar I would suggest writing on your wall calendar like you would a cheat. Be sure NOT to eat sugar on a daily basis even in the smallest amounts. Wean yourself slowly, over time, off of sugar if you need to.

Sugar suppresses the activity of our white blood cells, which makes us more susceptible to infectious disease (colds, the flu, and so forth) as well as cancer," explains Dr. Perricone in a recent article. Plus, sugar overload can cause collagen fibers to lose their strength, making skin "more vulnerable to sun damage, wrinkles, and sagging," he adds.

Low carb/Low sugar fruits and vegetables

- Artichokes
- Asparagus
- Berries
- Bok choy
- Broccoli
- Brussels sprouts
- Cauliflower
- Celery
- cucumber
- Kale
- Leafy greens like lettuce, spinach, kale, collards and swiss chard
- Mushrooms
- Radishes
- Spinach, Swiss Chard
- Tomatoes (nightshade alert)

Vegetables with a higher, naturally occurring, amount of sugar. It is the naturally occurring sugars in these foods that makes them high carb foods to avoid or at least limit portions if trying to lose or maintain weight:

Beets
Corn (grain)
Green peas
Legumes
Pumpkin
Shallots
Sweet Potato

According to sugar-and-sweetener-guide.com the following is a list of **natural sweeteners** that do NOT register on the Glycemic Index:
(I purposely did not include artificial sweeteners)

Brazzein
Curculin
Glycyrrhizin
Luo han guo
Miraculin
Monellin
Pentadin
Stevia: the most widely recognized here in the United States
Thaumatin

Using Stevia for the occasional sweetener is perfectly fine but don't use this to spoil your sweet tooth. The brain just knows you are eating something that taste sweet and does not differentiate between a healthy sweet and an unhealthy sweet. Indulging in sweet tasting foods, even with the use of Stevia, will make it hard to resist the bad sweets like candy, pies and donuts. When doing the 45 Day Palate Cleanse I suggest avoiding all sweet tasting foods in order to tame your sweet tooth.

After the 45 day cleanse if you feel the need to occasionally use a sweetener you can sweeten foods or beverages with fruits, raw honey or stevia. If you use stevia be sure to check the label of ingredients as some have fillers that you don't want. SweetLeaf Natural Stevia Sweetener is one of the choices that do not use fillers.

Some people will argue that carrots and other vegetables have a higher amount of sugar. Unless you are diabetic or have some other physical condition that the doctor as instructed you to stay away from foods with even the sugar content of carrots I would argue that for the otherwise healthy person, even someone trying to lose weight, carrots are fine. For one thing most people do not eat a pound of carrots a day. Or at least they should not.
Look at twofoods.com and compare carrots to a potato. A carrot has just 10 carbs (sugar is carbs) while a potato has 96 carbs. A potato can spike your blood sugar levels just like pure sugar due to the carb count.

A banana versus a cup of carrot sticks, say as a choice for a snack, is also interesting: the banana has 22 carbs versus just 9 if you choose the carrots.

Certainly compared to cakes and cookies, vegetables are a better choice. Even the high sugared, high carb sweet potato:

According to twofoods.com

Baked or Mashed Sweet Potato (with just butter only): 20 carbs
The equivalent amount of Oatmeal cookies: 68 carbs

I eat an unsweetened carrot puree that I make myself most mornings for breakfast but I do not eat sweets and desserts. I eat the occasional apple and the very occasional sweet potato, whipped like mashed potatoes, baked or diced in a stew. I have raw honey periodically as well. This compared to years ago when I use to eat pop tarts, muffins, cold cereal and waffles with syrup. At the time I felt I ate a fairly healthy diet as I never ate desserts. But, between my choice of breakfast foods and the occasional donut at work functions and other get togethers I was definitely consuming too much sugar.

Add the high carbs to that type of diet like baked potatoes, French fries, breads, breading, bottled dressings and sauces, juice, and cola's and I was really eating an overall unhealthy diet and I didn't even know it. Not only did I not eat desserts, but I did not bake, I did not eat candy, I hardly snacked, and even though I drank cola I was not an over-consuming fanatic about it. I maybe drank one single serve bottle a day with my lunch.

44 DAIRY

Dairy provides calcium but studies have shown it to also cause inflammation in the body. Although many people consume dairy without experiencing any problems, there are those who have a sensitivity or allergy to dairy, and those who want to avoid dairy because it causes inflammation resulting in painful flares among other symptoms. See Chapter 4 on Calcium for non-dairy food choices to get the recommended daily allowance of calcium. Some have to avoid casein altogether while others find they have a tolerance on occasion in small portions.

Casein allergy and lactose intolerance

Casein is the active ingredient in dairy products that causes the problem for most people. Being sensitive or allergic to Casein and being Lactose intolerant are two different things.

You are lactose intolerant when your body does not make a specific enzyme called lactase. This can make you feel very uncomfortable after consuming dairy.

Dairy products containing less protein and more fat, such as real butter and cream, contain very little casein. Clarified butter, or ghee, contains no casein at all. Many find they can eat Real Butter and whole fat cream, in limited amounts, on occasion without experiencing any problems. If you do find you are experiencing bad side effects from real butter or cream then simply avoid them all together.

Dairy products include, but are not limited to:

- Cow's Milk
- Yogurt
- Ice cream
- Powdered milk
- Cheese
- Kefir
- Cream cheese
- Sour cream
- Parmesan cheese

Eggs are not a dairy product even though we find them in the dairy department of the grocery store. Dairy products come from cows milk and products made from cows milk. Eggs come from chickens, not cows. That is why eggs are a good source of protein. All animals and animal by-products are generally good sources of protein.

If you are hypothyroid and avoiding soy products, be careful when replacing milk products. Read your labels and be sure you are not replacing the dairy product with a soy product. There are some new Almond Milk Yogurt products on the market that I found contain soy milk blended with the almond milk.

Always do what works for you!

If something bothers you after eating you need to add that food to your Banned Foods List and avoid it. If you find you can consume a food in small, occasional quantities then keep a wall calendar where you can jot down when that food is consumed so you are sure to not have it too often. We are each going to have our own unique experience with various foods, especially dairy, and need to pay attention to our bodies reaction to enjoy our best health possible.

A good alternative to dairy milk is Almond Milk. Be sure to choose Unflavored Original. This will be much more versatile in the kitchen and you can always add vanilla or chocolate for those occasional recipes that you use vanilla flavored almond milk.

45 NIGHTSHADES

There are deadly nightshade plants that we know to avoid. Toxic plants like Scopolamine. But there are also foods we have been consuming for centuries that are in that same nightshade family. While they may not cause the delirium and hallucinations of the deadly nightshade plants they can, after time, compound in our bodies, and cause symptoms for some people with autoimmune diseases like arthritis as well as inflammatory diseases and conditions such as those who suffer from migraine headaches.

Nightshades have Lectins, molecules that can attach to the walls of the intestine causing health issues in the gut to flare, joint pain and swelling for those with arthritis and more.

Let's be clear that there is no scientific evidence that nightshades cause autoimmune diseases. Only that it can make your symptoms worse. Many have found great relief by omitting all foods that cause inflammation and flares; one being foods that are in the nightshade family.

Foods in the nightshade family:

- Tomatoes and Tomatillos
- Eggplant
- White, gold and red potatoes
- Goji berries
- Peppers: all peppers (for example: bell peppers, chili peppers, paprika, tamales, cayenne. Just to name A few. (All peppers)
- Pimento
- Spices like paprika, cayenne, red pepper, taco seasoning, chili seasonings
- Ketchup, hot sauce, spaghetti sauce, sloppy joe mix
- Tobacco (although not a food it is consumed into the body)

Often questioned, but these are NOT nightshades:

- Black pepper
- Blueberries
- Cumin
- Mushrooms
- Onions
- Sweet potatoes and yams

But if you find any of these foods bother you in any way simply avoid eating them.

Tobacco, a plant, is also a part of the nightshade family and should be avoided if you are avoiding nightshades or want to do an elimination diet of nightshades to see if your symptoms lessen after getting nightshades out of your system.

As with any elimination diet to find out your tolerance level, you must first go at least 45 consecutive days without any foods from the food group(s) you are concerned or curious about; i.e.: dairy, soy, nightshades, grains, sugar, or gluten.

The reason for the 45 consecutive days is that these foods have compounded in the body over the last 20 years or so and it can take up to 45 days to rid them completely from the body before you will notice relief. Once you have gone 45 consecutive days you should assess yourself; Are you still experiencing symptoms?

If many, or all of your symptoms have diminished or lessened, you know something you stopped eating was causing your symptoms to worsen. Now to find out if you have a tolerance for any of the foods you eliminated.

Each person can have a different experience, Some have zero tolerance while others can tolerate some foods in small amounts on a limited basis.

Re-introduce foods one food at a time; to be eaten daily for at least 3 consecutive days to see if your symptoms return.

For example re-introduce just real butter. Eat in normal portions for 3 consecutive days. Assess your symptoms, if any. If any symptoms return stop eating the butter. Now you can move onto another food. Exercise some patience and remember that this does take time but that it will all be worth it!

46 GLUTEN

Gluten is found in all wheat products.

I have talked to several people who did not understand what gluten or wheat products are. Of course, if you are not sensitive to gluten you would have no reason for researching and understanding it either. For those of you new to learning what wheat products are I hope to clear up some of the misconceptions I have found some people to have on this topic.

Wheat products are foods made from wheat. This includes while bread and not just whole wheat bread. I have also talked with people who thought just white bread had gluten but whole wheat bread did not. Both are made from wheat and both have gluten.

If the ingredient label states: flour, unbleached whole wheat flour or bleached flour then that product is made from wheat.

All gluten products are processed foods. If you are leaning toward eating a diet that is unprocessed fresh foods you will by default eliminate gluten from your diet. Fresh fruits and vegetables as well as meats and seafood do not contain gluten. Please note that prepared frozen dinners with meats and vegetables generally DO have gluten; but they are processed foods.

Most fresh foods do not have labels and are not in boxes. Get your meat and seafood from the meat and seafood department and the bulk of your vegetables from the produce department. FRESH FOODS THAT ARE NOT PROCESSED OR PRE-COOKED.

Prepared and or pre-cooked foods are all processed. As you move more toward eating fresh, unprocessed foods you will not have to read all those labels! There are certainly some processed foods that are not OVERLY processed and suitable on a fresh unprocessed foods diet. Foods like Olive oil, Raw unfiltered Apple Cider Vinegar, canned artichokes (not marinated varieties), and there are even a few canned vegetables like sauerkraut and Libby green beans.

All gluten foods are also high carb foods and gluten is known to cause inflammation in some people.

Bread
Breading
Cereal
Crackers
Flour Pasta
Rye
Barley
Beer (Wines and distilled liquors do not contain gluten)
Malted milk
Malt vinegar
Graham crackers
Saltines
Pretzels
Pie crust and pizza crust
Panko
Stuffing and dressings
Processed, prepared gravy, sauces, dressings and soups generally have flour as a thickener
Flour tortillas
Seasoning packets: check the label
Some supplements contain gluten. Read your labels.

Even gluten free flour, bread, pasta, cereal, crackers, etcetera are high carb foods. Not only that, they are processed foods and should be eaten sparingly if at all. Gluten free does not mean low carb. Those of you avoiding grains and/or soy products will also want to avoid the "gluten free" **processed** foods because in the absence of using wheat flour these products use grain flours like Rice flour or Soy flour.

My own diet is virtually gluten free, dairy free, soy free, nightshade free and grain free. I say virtually because I find I can tolerate small, occasional portions of a gluten free flour (generally a rice flour) but I don't make cakes or brownies. I'm talking about a tablespoon once a month or so to make a sauce or gravy. I find I can also tolerate the smidgeon of grated parmesan cheese (tiny sprinklings) on foods perhaps once a month. Some people cannot even tolerate the tiniest amounts and if you are one of those you should leave those out of any recipe.

An alternative for making a roux or slurry to thicken a sauce or gravy is Arrowroot. Arrowroot looks and behaves much like cornstarch but it is a plant and not a grain or gluten. Or pureed vegetables also works! Puree with broth, almond milk or water.

47 GRAINS

A list of the common grains:

Wheat (gluten)
Rice
Corn
Oats

If you are trying to lose weight filling up on whole grains will most likely not help. A great online tool is a site called twofoods.com Suppose you are having dinner and have the choice of brown rice or cauliflower (riced or chopped and then sautéed) as a side dish.

Comparing these two foods on twofoods.com

1 cup of brown rice has:
- Calories: 216
- Carbs: 44

Whereas one cup of cauliflower has:
- Calories: 25
- Carbs: 5.5

One cup of cauliflower may not fill you up like one cup of brown rice. You can double your serving of cauliflower and still be consuming half the calories and carbs of the rice, or you could choose a second vegetable like a salad, green beans, or asparagus.

48 TOBACCO

There is nothing positive to say about tobacco. It has no redeeming qualities at all. No nutritional value either.

I was a smoker for 20 years and quit when I was age 40. In retrospect I cannot believe I smoked at all. Quitting is one of the best things I've ever done for myself and those around me.

Tobacco is also a nightshade plant meaning it can trigger painful flares in those vulnerable to stiffness and joint or muscle pain.

49 CONSTIPATION

One of the most uncomfortable conditions to live with is chronic constipation. If you have been to the doctor and the advice your doctor has given you is not helping I encourage you to try changing your diet.

Many find that gluten, dairy and grains actually cause their constipation. If eating high fiber whole grains (glutens/grains) haven't offered you any relief try vegetables with fiber. To get you *going* try eating a dark green leafy every day while also avoiding glutens, grains and dairy 100% for at least 45 consecutive days.

Great sources of vegetable fiber: (and a few fruits that are lower in sugar)

- Artichokes
- Almonds, Pecans and walnuts
- Blackberries (fresh only)
- Broccoli
- Brussels Sprouts
- *Flaxseed, ground
- Green Beans (cooked from fresh)
- Green peas
- Raspberries (fresh only)
- Spinach
- Sweet Potato (baked, with the skin) (high carb food alert)

*Ground flaxseed provides your body with the benefits of both soluble and insoluble fibers, whole flax seeds only provides you with insoluble fiber due to its outer shell. Flaxseed is a true plant and not a gluten or grain.

See chapter 11 on Fiber for more information

If you are looking for a supplement to help get back to regular bowel movements you might try 100mg Magnesium Citrate after your evening meal. There are different kinds of Magnesium and most find relief with this one.

50 RESTLESS LEG SYNDROME AND RINGING OF THE EARS

In the past 10 years there has been an upswing of individuals looking for some relief of RLS (restless leg syndrome) and ringing of the ears. I too suffer from both of these. It started about 12 years ago. It was after I was able to find some relief for myself that I started talking to my clients about their own experiences. Here is what I found:

While not all people found relief with this method many did, including myself.

Triggers for RLS and Ringing of the Ears both seem to be consumption of the following for two or more days in a row. Once a week, on portion, most could handle without triggering symptoms. It was only after two or more days in a row that the suffering would begin again. Avoiding these two or more days in a row, or avoiding completely for some, and most found they did not have a re-occurrence of restless leg or ringing in the ears.

- Citrus: citrus fruits, juice, citric acid found in processed foods and OTC vitamins, tums and other foods and drinks.
- Pain Relievers: acetaminophen and ibuprofen
- OTC meds like sleep aids

51 CANDIDA, YEAST INFECTIONS AND ATHLETES FOOT

Candida is a fungus that lives inside the body, and when out of control can cause painful rashes on and inside the body in the form of yeast infections, athletes foot and even inside the mouth and on the belly. When out of control Candida can cause other health problems like digestive issues, bloating, fatigue, and brain fog. It can sometimes reveal itself as a red rash when you sweat. Common areas are the neck, chest and stomach.

Candida is made worse by sugar and foods that are broken down into sugars by the body like grains, including gluten. Some are so sensitive to sugar they need to avoid even healthy sugars like fruit and raw honey before seeing their symptoms subside.

A Candida diet really can make a significant difference in your quality of life if you have ongoing issues with yeast infections, athletes foot or candida inside the body. The bulk of your foods should be focused on exactly what we have talked about in this book. Meats, seafood and vegetables. Non starchy vegetables making up the bulk of your food choices. Stay away from foods known to cause inflammation like sugar, dairy, gluten and grains until you have your symptoms under control and feel better. Then try just one food, small portions at a time, to find out your tolerance level (how much and how often you can consume a specific food before triggering a symptom). I recommend doing a search for candida and learning as much as you can. Other lifestyle choices that may help:

- After bathing always shower off. Look at it this way, you wouldn't wash a dish and not rinse it.

- After showering be sure to thoroughly dry your skin. *All of your skin* but particularly your feet, between the toes, your intimate areas, under your arms, and under flaps of skin that are not necessarily exposed to air as easily like under the breasts.

- If you have a history of yeast infections and you douche, stop. At least for the 45 day elimination diet period. You should find that you do not need to douche at all. The only time you should douche is under the direction of your doctor.

- Avoid foods that are known to trigger a flare: sugar (even natural occurring sugars), carbohydrates like flours, grains, dairy, and legumes, mushrooms (fungi), dried spices and dried teas can also be a problem for some who are especially sensitive. Be mindful to purchase only fresh products and do not use after 6 months.

52 SLEEP

It all starts with getting a good night's sleep.

It seems many of us are having a problem sleeping. This is concerning as it can potentially increase the number of people seeking over-the-counter or even prescription medication in our effort to get some rest.

We have all read the list of suggestions on how to get a good night's sleep:

Dark room
Warm bath
No electronics

These suggestions do help to relax the mind. There is a difference in mental tiredness and physically being tired. It is my own opinion that mental tiredness causes interruptions in our sleep while physical tiredness promotes sleep. Caffeine is also a problem for those that are more sensitive to caffeine.

The most natural and direct path to getting a good night's sleep is to be more active during the day so that you are physically tired and it helps to cut down on your caffeine. Set a cut-off time early in the day like 10am or omit caffeine all together.

I did my own unofficial study with me and 10 of my clients a few years ago. We all had office jobs (not labor intense jobs) and we all drank coffee or caffeinated colas every day. We all limited our caffeine to just one cup of coffee before 9am and no caffeinated colas and we all increased our daily standing activities by 3 hours a day. About half of us started sleeping without taking any sleep medication and those who did also reported that they felt the quality of sleep was better; as if they relaxed more while sleeping.

Then we omitted all caffeine while continuing with our commitment to at least 3 hours of standing activities and exercise per day. All but one of us found we fell asleep within minutes of going to bed without taking anything at all and we slept through the night. We also found we too felt more rested in the morning as though our muscles had relaxed more than usual.

Starting a daily exercise regimen for yourself is a great start. Try stretching (or your back exercises) in the morning. This should take anywhere from 15 to 30 minutes. After lunch or after supper walk 30-60 minutes. There's another 30-60 minutes (subtotal: 45-90 minutes). For the remainder of the time find things to do every day that keeps you on your feet and moving as much as possible.

- Fold laundry standing instead of sitting
- Stand every time you check your phone
- Stand as you look through the mail
- Move items you use daily to the top shelf where you have to use a step stool and reach for it and some items to the bottom shelves forcing you to squat and stand back up.
- Shower every day (standing!)
- Make your bed every day
- Sweep the tile areas of your house daily
- Stand every time you take a phone call
- Stand when preparing foods: I see a lot of people sitting while they chop vegetables!
- Make it a habit that every time you go to the restroom that you also do 3 or 4 "touch your toe" repetitions.

53 ARTHRITIS

They symptoms of arthritis; joint pain, stiffness, and swelling of joints is caused by inflammation so it makes sense that avoiding foods that are known to cause inflammation may give you some much needed relief.

Many people scoff at the idea that changing ones diet can actually help when doctors are prescribing such powerful medicines as treatment. I mean, if it were as simple as not eating tomatoes wouldn't the doctor tell me?

Well, not necessarily. For one thing, as hard as it is to believe, doctors really are not schooled in nutrition and how it may negatively impact the body. They are schooled in medicine that is used to react and treat a medical problem once it appears. Not in nutritional habits as a way of prevention or as a way to control symptoms of disease like arthritis or other autoimmune diseases.

The doctors I have spoken to and worked with through the years also tell me they have lost patients after suggesting to them an anti-inflammatory diet. Patients just aren't on board yet. We ARE getting there though.

I have to admit I too did not believe what I was reading. Perhaps it was my resistance to change or just me not wanting to give up my tomatoes! Not sure, but after 8 years of suffering even with doctor prescribed Plaquenil and Hydrocodone, and more and more symptoms and problems adding on year after year I finally decided it certainly would not hurt me to give this "diet" thing a try. The first time was a feeble attempt. I went just one week without tomatoes only. I continued to eat other nightshades, gluten, dairy and sugar. And really, just one week is not a full-fledged effort.

About six months after the first attempt I again found myself just fed up with the pain and feeling bad and decided if I was going to see if this worked that I really had to commit to it for at least 2 months, about 60 consecutive days. 100% commitment. No Gluten. No Dairy. No Grains. No Nightshades.

I started a countdown on the calendar; 60, 59, 58, ... Then I would mess up eating something I shouldn't have and so I would just start over the following day: 60, 59, 58. It took me approximately one year to finally successfully go 60 days without cheating at all. I noticed as soon as 2 weeks a subtle difference. At 30 days even better and at 45 days so much better that I did not want to turn back. By my 60 days I was astounded that I felt even better than at the 45 day mark.

It was astounding enough to me that this really worked and I no longer found the need to take pain killers anymore but there were other benefits I was not expecting.

My entire life I had dealt with an ongoing depression that came and went. Sometimes it came and stayed way too long and was quite heavy. I realized after four or five months that I had not had a bout with my depression in a while. Then one day I cheated and had some gluten. I think it was the bun on a hamburger. The next morning I woke up with a terrible bout of depression. It was awful. It took about 3 days to go away. Three days of me back on my diet strictly.

I also noticed I was sleeping better. My allergies had dissipated so much so that I no longer needed my Claritin-D: congestion was gone. I had lived nearly 20 years suffering with severe congestion and allergies and now, suddenly just gone with a change of my diet. No more money spent on decongestants and nasal sprays.

For years I had a regular unknown pain in my chest. No more.

Inflammation in the body can affect you in so many ways!

I have learned that if I want to join the family at a Mexican or Italian restaurant known for including glutens and nightshades that I make sure I am strictly adhering to my diet leading up to the event and then the day of the event I take some over the counter pain pills, just one dose is usually fine. I also make sure to stick to my diet in the days following. This way I am not compounding the inflammatory foods over the period of a few days. Doing so will allow the buildup in the body which causes the trigger of symptoms. I also know to expect the possibility of waking up depressed. There is great comfort in knowing what triggered it though. Knowing it will only last a couple of days and will go away!

These foods do not cause depression or arthritis or other autoimmune and inflammatory conditions. That is why a large portion of the population can eat them without having any issues. But for those of us with health conditions the diet can be a very effective tool to not only ease symptoms but stop them.

Just as important as diet to easing symptoms of arthritis is exercise. I wanted to share with you two good sources of reliable information:

- bones.nih.gov/health-info/bone-health/exercise/exercise-your-bone-health (exercise and bone health)
- mayoclinic.org/diseases-conditions/arthritis/in-depth/arthritis/art-20047971 (more about exercise and joint health)

The take-a-way is that even though it may be challenging to get started it can be very beneficial and life changing to start. Even if you start with just 5 minutes a day most find they very quickly are able to increase that steadily over the course of just a month to 30 minutes a day.

Exercising reduces joint pain, strengthens bones, increases strength, stamina and flexibility and combats fatigue. Just start where you are and build on that.

Weight bearing exercises are your best choice. If you have knee pain keeping you up at night and down during the day walking (a weight bearing exercise) can make all the difference. Most find once they work their way to at least 20-30 minutes a day the knee pain literally disappears and they have no more need for pain medications. Stay away from stairs except for the occasional and not until your knee pain has subsided. If you live in a two story house consider moving to a one story or to a room downstairs. Just one more way to care for your knees. Most find once they have their knee pain under control they can use stairs occasionally but use on a daily basis causes problems.

Find a nearby park, hiking trail, walk around the block or better yet get a treadmill so that darkness or inclement weather wont hinder your ability to walk every single day. Go outside as often as you can and use your treadmill as a backup.

Another part of the body that can benefit from weight bearing exercises is the spine. Laying on your back, on the floor, a hard surface is where you should start. The weight of your body while lying flat and straight, every day will go a long way to alleviating back pain. From there do some back exercises to keep your back pain completely gone.

Doing these exercises daily (at least 6 days per week) can help some of the most painful backs. Try it for at least one month, 6 days a week to see if they help you. Talk with your physician to make sure these are safe for you to perform.

The bridge:

1. Lay on the floor. Arms at your side and knees up.

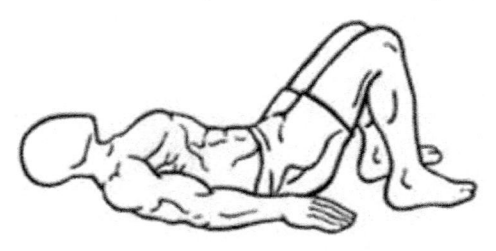

2. Lift your buttocks to create a bridge pose. Hold for a count of 8. Then slowly lower yourself back to the original position on the floor as in picture one (1). Repeat this 8 times every day. First thing in the morning is the best time as it will stretch your back before you start your day.

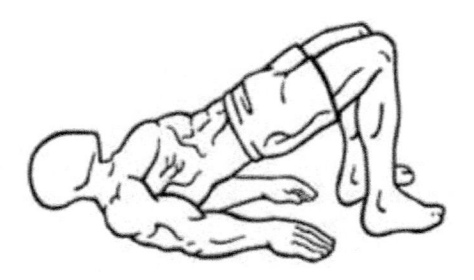

Side knee rolls:

Still on the floor with your knees pulled up and your back flat on the floor as in picture one of the bridge exercise, extend your arms straight out and allow both knees to gently fall to one side at the waist. Hold for a count of 8 and then return to the original position. Hold for a count of 8 and then allow the knees to gently fall to the opposite side, also holding for a count of 8 before returning to the original position. Your goal is to work up to being able to do 8 repetitions of this exercise six (6) days a week.

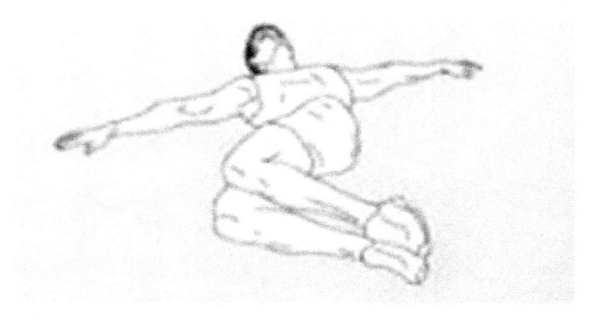

3. While on the floor touch your toes!

   Start by lying flat on your back. Hands to your side.

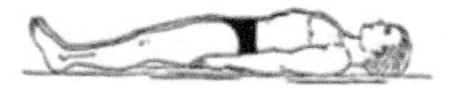

4. Sit up and reach to touch your toes and hold for a count of 8.

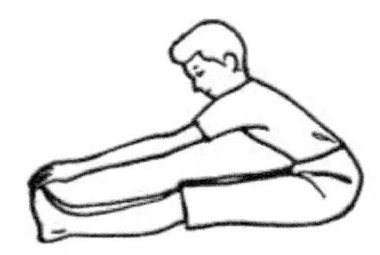

   Release and return to lying down flat on the floor position. Count to 8.

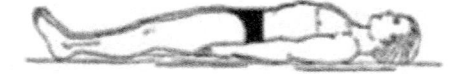

Sit back up and gently reach to touch your toes again. Hold for a count of 8.

Your goal is to be able to do this repetition 8 times. This is a great stretch for the lower back and by lying back down flat on the floor as your starting position between each rep makes for a good strengthening exercise for your core or abdominal area.

Touching your toes from the standing position will also stretch your lower back but is also a good stretch for your legs and ankles.

Start in a standing position. Hands at your side.

Stretch your arms straight above your head before slowly bending over to touch your toes. Hold this for a count of 8. Stretching your arms up as if reaching:

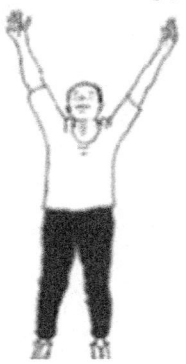

When you bend over to touch your toes hold for a count of 8 before standing back up. Your eventual goal is 8 repetitions six times a week.

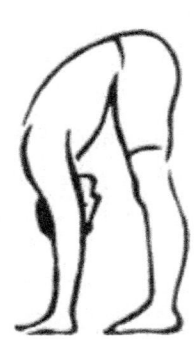

Floor exercises are also a great opportunity to keep you flexible and strong enough to get down on the floor and back up off the floor. Your goal is to be able to do this unassisted. If at first you need to use furniture or even another person to safely get up then absolutely do! But, your goal is to get down and back up unaided.

For younger healthy people you should know that the reason this is important for even **you** to know is because if you want to be able to continue doing something as you grow older you must continue to do it on a regular basis.

The biggest reason older people cannot get up when they fall down is because at some point they stopped getting on the floor and getting back up. Not because of injury or illness. Do this daily as a matter of exercise even if you don't need to get on the floor. This will keep you agile.

Staying strong and at a healthy weight by walking, and doing floor exercises among other activities will keep help your balance and stability.

Why is this so important?

According to the CDC more than 300,000 older people fall each year. About 95% of those result in a fracture or broken bone. Even those who do not fracture or break a bone, many find they cannot get up without help. For older folks who live alone or with another older person not in the best of health this could be problematic if you cannot get to a phone for help.

Falls are preventable and again, aging in and of itself is not the reason we can't get back up. It's because we stopped doing it! If you stopped doing it because getting down onto the floor and back up by yourself became difficult that is actually all the more reason to change your diet and start a daily exercise program so that it will become easy again. Your quality of life greatly diminishes if you allow yourself to end up in the recliner all day dependent on someone else.

For those of you suffering with joint pain in your hands and fingers keep a soft touch fabric cold compress (ice pack) nearby. I keep one in a insulated lunch bag and take it with me to the office and also to bed at night. Put a small hard ice pack in the insulated bag to help keep your cold compress cold when not in use. I find squeezing the soft cold compress straight out of the freezer every morning for a few minutes helps the swelling and stiffness I usually wake up with. I use the blue cold compress easily found just about anywhere: Ace Large Reusable Cold Compress Soft Touch fabric by 3M.

54 HYPOTHYROID

Hyperthyroid is an over active thyroid [hence the hyper-]
Hypothyroid is an under active thyroid.

You and your doctor are the best source of information but from my own experience coupled with my clients input, classes I have taken and studies I have read I will say this:

Avoid soy products. See the chapter on soy.

A suggested supplement:

Selenium has antioxidant properties, which may help your body fight off illnesses. It also helps maintain the immune system and regulate thyroid function.

Biotin for dry, brittle hair, skin and nails. 5000 to 10,000 capsule per day. Found in the supplement and vitamin isle of most any store.
Some symptoms that may want you to consider avoiding soy to see if you might feel better and seek a thyroid test from your doctor:

- Thinning and frizzy hair for no other reason
- Mood swings
- Bouts of extreme anger
- Sensitive to cold or heat
- Constipation for no other reason
- Unexplained weight gain
- Extreme fatigue and tiredness
- Brittle nails
- Dry skin
- unusual high cholesterol results
- Irregular menstrual periods

Eating a healthy diet based on unprocessed foods and staying as active as possible can go a long way to feeling back to normal. Speak to your doctor about having your thyroid checked if you suspect thyroid dysfunction.

Weight gain is often a big complaint, or rather the inability to lose weight with this condition. I will tell you that what has worked in the past may not work now. It does not mean you have to starve or go hungry in order to maintain a heathy weight. Change to non-starchy low carb foods like we highlight here in this book: meats, seafood and low carb vegetables as 99% of your diet and you will be on your way to your normal weight again. Watch your fruits and remember that packaged gluten free products are still high carb foods such as gluten free breads, cereals, flours, etc. They are simply gluten free but not low carb.

Do a comparison of wheat flour and rice flour. Rice flour is most commonly the gluten free alternative. When comparing be sure you are comparing the same serving size. I did a quick look at twofoods.com to compare wheat flour and rice flour and noticed the wheat flour carbs were based on just a ¼ cup size serving yet the rice flour was based on 100 grams (1/2 cup).

55 ALCOHOL

Which alcoholic beverages have gluten and which do not?

Alcoholic beverages that are gluten free:

- Wine
- Distilled Spirits
- Tequila from the Agave plant

All others are either glutens, made from wheat and others, like most Vodka is made from potatoes which is a nightshade.

Some other warnings about alcohol consumption:

- If you are hypothyroid you should know that alcohol can wreak havoc on the thyroid and on hormones regulated by the thyroid. If you drink at all, drink within limitations.

- Alcohol and Gout. If you have gout you have probably been warned by your doctor that an attack can be brought on by purine rich foods. Beer is high in purines.

- Alcohol can lessen the effect of some medications, supplements and even absorption of some nutrients of foods you eat.

- To find out what part alcohol may be playing in triggering symptoms for you I suggest avoiding it entirely during the 45 day elimination diet and reintroduce one type, one serving at a time to find out your tolerance level: Tolerance level (how much and how often you can consume a specific food before triggering a symptom if at all).

56 SOY

If you have been diagnosed with hypothyroid your doctor has most likely warned you to not consume soy products:

- Soy sauce
- Soybeans
- Soy milk
- Soybean oil (vegetable oil) Read the label. Also found in many cans of tuna and chicken.
- Tofu
- Edamame beans

Even if you have not been diagnosed with thyroid the problem with thyroid is that unless you bring it up the doctor will most likely not test your thyroid function. Even when they do, the doctor has a range of "normal" and if you fall within the range they will not give you a diagnosis or medication. The problem with this is that many people have symptoms with the slightest variance of their thyroid.

Some symptoms that may want you to consider avoiding soy to see if you might feel better:

Thinning and frizzy hair for no other reason
Mood swings
Bouts of extreme anger
Sensitive to cold or heat
Constipation for no other reason
Unexplained weight gain
Extreme fatigue and tiredness
Brittle nails
Dry skin
unusual high cholesterol results
Irregular menstrual periods

Eating a healthy diet based on unprocessed foods and staying as active as possible can go a long way to feeling back to normal. Speak to your doctor about having your thyroid checked if you suspect thyroid dysfunction.

Always consult with your physician before adding supplements. Especially if you are currently on prescription medications or have been diagnosed with a health issue.

Supplement Suggestion for the thyroid:

For dry brittle nails, dry skin and dry thinning hair my physician suggested 10,000 mcg Biotin. I tried 5000 mcg a day first and after 3 months of virtually no change tried the 10,000 mcg / day with success.

Selenium 200 mcg either daily or every other day

Follow directions on supplements just like you would prescription medication.

57 BREATHING CLEAN AIR

Oxygen is one of those elements often overlooked when talking about maintaining a healthier body. Oxygen is needed by your brain as well as all cells of the body. Breathing in clean air is never more important than to counteract damage done by pollution, second hand smoke, fumes and allergens.

You don't necessarily need to sit down and meditate daily, although that does have its benefits, but you should be mindful of the breathes you take and the air you are inhaling. When in an environment you know has the cleanest air possible get into the habit of taking some deep breaths through the nose, exhaling through the mouth. Toxins picked up throughout the day will be expelled in that exhale. The clean air acts as a sort of filter but you must make sure the air in your home is as clean as possible.

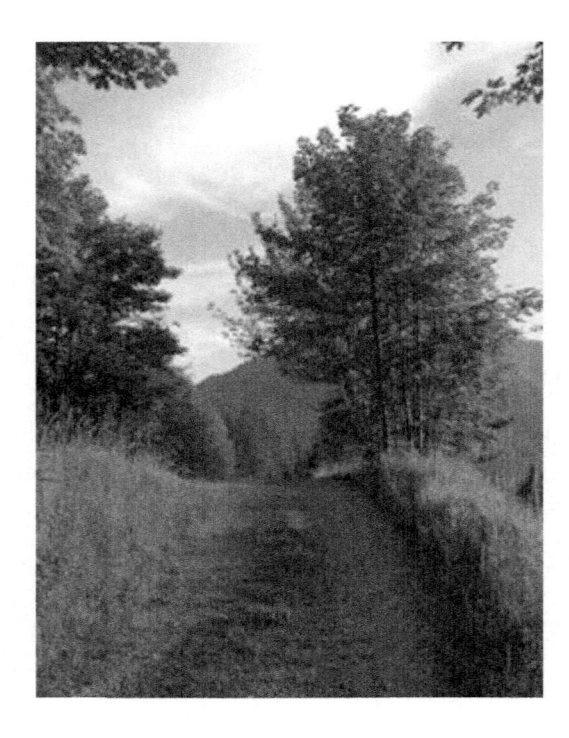

Fresh clean outdoor air is best.

But don't forget the air in your home. Be sure your home is free of:

- Scented products like cleaning supplies and perfumes
- Aerosol's like Lysol spray and air fresheners
- Cigarette smoke

Scented products, cleaning supply scents and fumes, aerosols and cigarette smoke can trigger Asthma and Allergies.

Fresh clean air has its health benefits:

- Cleans the lungs and improves lung function
- Releases toxins from the body
- Increased energy
- Helps the brain to function with more clarity
- Aids in digestion. Taking a walk outside, even a short one, after each meal can be very beneficial!
- Polluted air outside and inside the home causes the body to work harder which can result in higher blood pressure and increased heart rate.

Deep breathes of fresh, clean air increases Serotonin. Serotonin is worth reading up on! Serotonin does many things for the body, one is mood balance. The very reason it is suggested that we stop and take deep breaths when we feel frustrated, angry or anxious. Also good for depression and just feeling overall happier.

This is one of the main reasons people shout the benefits of daily meditation and how it's changed their lives. During mediation it is suggested that you take in deep breathes through the nose, that are to be exhaled out the mouth.

58 THE IMPORTANCE OF ABSORPTION

The importance of absorbing nutrients from your foods and the active ingredients from your medications and supplements cannot be stressed enough, and yet seldom discussed.

Many dismiss the effectiveness of a food, medication, or vitamin without first making sure they are not hindering the body's ability to absorb what you need.

I started learning about this first hand while seeing an allergist. My seasonal allergies had turned into daily, year 'round allergies. My allergist prescribed Claritin D (this was in the 90s when you still needed a prescription). On my return visit 3 months later I told the doctor I had not seen much improvement, a little but not enough. He responded by telling me to give it another 3 months and if it was still not working for me then we would try something else.

Sometime over the next 3 months I read a magazine article that shared a study that showed when we do not take most medications with a **full glass of water** that our bodies are only absorbing approximately 20% of the active ingredient. That many patients complained of medications not working well but they were taking medications with just a sip of water, or taking them with cola, coffee, juice or no beverage at all. The study showed that the majority found remarkable improvement after they started taking medications, vitamins and supplements with a full glass of plain water.
Oh! That's interesting information. So I started taking my allergy medication with a full glass of plain water and nearly all of my symptoms subsided. It was remarkable to say the least. Such a small thing to do.

In the years to come I found we also need to make sure we are doing all we can to help our bodies not only absorb medications, vitamins, and supplements but also the nutrients provided in our foods.

The following will help in absorption:

- Chewing your food well
- Taking all medications, supplements and vitamins with at least 10 ounces of water unless otherwise instructed. Many people just take a "sip". Just enough to get it swallowed. Furthermore, many are taking with coffee, cola, juice, milk or other beverages or none at all!
- Follow the directions on the label. If your supplement says to take on an empty stomach you should do that (with water!) If it states to take *with a meal* then take the supplement or medication *during* a meal (a few bites in). If it says *after or before a meal* then you should take it exactly as it states. Following the directions literally will give you the best benefits.
- Drink sips water with your meals to help your body absorb the nutrients in your foods. Forego other beverages.
- Healthy fats can increase your absorption of fat-soluble vitamins including vitamins A, D, E and K. Refer to chapter 79 *Healthy Fats* for a list of food sources.
- Do not store supplements, vitamins, prescriptions, or over-the-counter medication in the bathroom. Nor do you want to store them in a cupboard in the kitchen near the stove. The humidity of the bathroom and the heat from the stove can break down the active ingredients. Store in a dry, cool, dark cupboard. I keep mine on the shelf of my bedroom closet in a plastic bin and my pillbox that I fill each week inside a desk drawer in my home office.

59 RDA quick glance Table

NUTRIENT	MALE	FEMALE
Biotin	30 mcg	30 mcg
Calcium	1000 mg	1200 mg
Carbohydrates	150 grams	120 grams
Choline	550 mg	550 mg
Chromium	35 mcg	25 mcg
Copper	900 mcg	900 mcg

NUTRIENT	MALE	FEMALE	
Fiber	25 G	25 G	
Folate	400 mcg	400 mcg	
Iodine	150 mcg	150 mcg	
Iron	9 mg	9-18 mg	Women still menstruating: 18 mg/day Women after menopause: 9 mg/day
Isoflavones	25 g	25 g	
Magnesium	400 mg	320 mg	

NUTRIENT	MALE	FEMALE
Manganese	2 mg	2 mg
Omega-3	400 mcg	400 mcg
Pantothenic acid	5 mg	5 mg
Phosphorus	700 mg	700 mg
Potassium	1600 mg	1600 mg
Protein	56 G	46 G

NUTRIENT	MALE	FEMALE
Selenium	55 mcg	55 mcg
Sodium	1500 <	1500 <
Vitamin A	900 mcg	900 mcg
Thiamin Vitamin B1	1-2 mg	1-2 mg
Vitamin B12	2.4 mcg	2.4 mcg
Riboflavin—Vit B12	2.5 mg	1.8 mg

NUTRIENT	MALE	FEMALE	
Niacin vitamin B3	16 ng	14 g	
Vitamin B6	2 mg	1.5 mg	
Vitamin C	609-90 mg	60-90 mg	
Vitamin D	5 mcg	5 mcg	... Or 400—900 IU of Vit D—be sure to consider the foods you eat when tallying your total daily Vitamin D consumption.
Vitamin E	15 mg	15 mg	
Vitamin K	120 mcg	90 mcg	

60 HEALTH BENEFITS OF HERBS

Don't underestimate the health benefits of incorporating fresh herbs into your diet! Often ignored as a garnish, herbs are a great way to season your dishes with fresh, unprocessed foods.

Leafy herbs are also included in the leafy greens group (the healthiest vegetables you can eat). So toss them in your salads, add them to your sauces, dressings, make Salsa Verde and enjoy these fresh flavors!

61 basil
62 bay leaf
63 chives
64 cilantro
65 dill
66 lemongrass
67 mint
68 oregano
69 parsley
70 rosemary
71 sage
72 tarragon
73 thyme

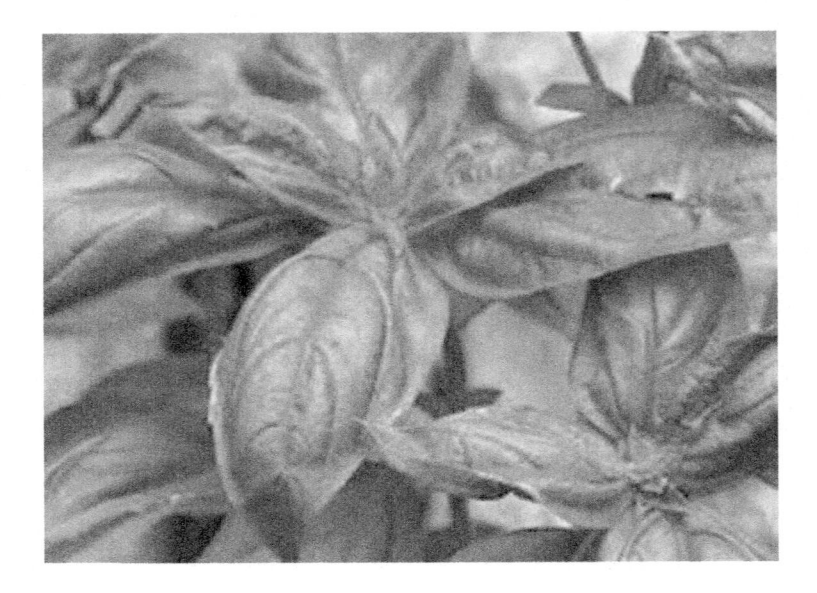

61 BASIL

Also known as St. Johns Wort

Lest we forget, fresh basil is a leafy green! Aromatic and full of flavor Basil should be a staple if it isn't already. Quite easy to grow in a container this is a great herb to grow yourself for year round use.

Heath benefits of fresh Basil:

Per each two (2) tablespoons:

- Vitamin K....................98%........RDA
- Manganese   12%........RDA
- Copper.......................09%........RDA
- Vitamin A....................06%
- Vitamin C....................05%

Source: whfoods.com

In a 2003 study published in the Journal of Microbiology Methods July 2003 issue, basil was shown to have anti-bacterial properties. A 2005 study suggests Basil has an anti-inflammatory benefit for those with conditions like rheumatoid arthritis and inflammatory bowel.

Known for it use in Italian dishes don't be shy about adding this to your salads, and try making a homemade pesto! Basil pesto is the perfect substitute for tomato sauce if you are avoiding nightshades.

Make an effort to incorporate more Fresh Basil into your diet.

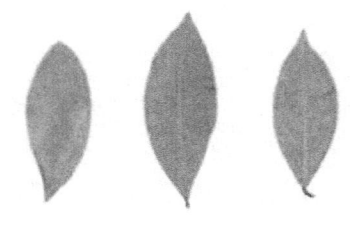

62 BAY LEAF

aka: Bay Leaves

Used for seasoning and flavoring but be sure to remove whole leaves prior to serving.

The Bay Leaf has many health benefits according to a varied health and medical establishments. According to organicfacts.net the bay leaf can:

- Improve digestion
- Settling upset stomachs for some (I find ginger root works best myself)
- Soothing IBS symptoms
- May help to lower levels of stress hormones in the body
- Aids in the absorption of other nutrients

Please note that there is a small portion of people allergic or sensitive to bay leaf. If you experience any negative side effects like stomach upset, headache or cramps after consuming something seasoning with bay leaf simply avoid it.

Standard use of Bay Leaves can deliver:

- Potassium......................10 mg
- Vitamin A......................02% RDA
- Vitamin C......................01% RDA

- Folic Acid......................01% RDA

...and according to nutrition-and-you.com an excellent source of minerals like copper, calcium, manganese selenium and zinc.

Have you tried a cup of Bay Leaf tea yet?

Add a leaf or two to a cup and a half of water, bring to a boil. Cover and allow to simmer for about 20 minutes (or steep). Add with another tea, spice or herb for additional flavor. Suggestions might be Chamomile, Green Tea, Mint Tea. I also will steep a cup to add to my Orange Pekoe Iced Tea.

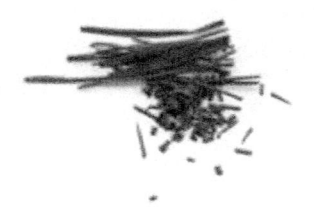

63 CHIVES

A delicate onion-y flavored stem of this flowering plant. A perennial that is drought tolerant and has beautiful purple blossoms. Easy peasy to grow in a container or herb garden.

For years I thought chives were only destined to land on the top of my baked potato in a restaurant. Then, I stopped eating baked potatoes and it sent me on a search for other uses of this beloved and time honored herb.

- Add them to your fresh salads
- Sprinkle atop your seafood
- Liven the top of your creamy soups and sauces
- Crown your deviled eggs
- Add as a edible garnish to your egg dishes like omelets, scrambled eggs and frittatas

I went to foodfacts.mercola.com to find out the health benefits we can derive from Chives. Per a two (2) tablespoon serving:

- 16%...RDA Vitamin K
- 01%.RDA Vitamin A

Chives are also a good source of your minerals like copper, iron, manganese and potassium.

Mercola cites Chives as having a combination of phytochemicals known to aid in digestion, prevent bad breath and perhaps assist in lowering blood pressure.

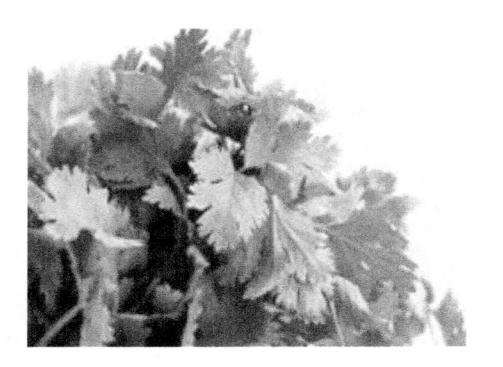

64 CILANTRO

Also known as Coriander but actually, not the same thing!
Same plant though so we are close. The leaf of the plant is known as cilantro. Whereas the seeds are Coriander. Cilantro, the leaf, is also referred to as Chinese Parsley.

Cilantro, a healthy leafy green, is known to deliver antioxidants, vitamins and some fiber. 4 Grams, or a quarter of a cup has:

- 21mg................Potassium
- 5%........RDA.......Vitamin A
- 1%........RDA.......Vitamin C
- .1 grams of fiber
- And Vitamin K

I encourage you to do a search for cilantro recipes! Not just a garnish. My most commonly used recipe is Salsa Verde which I first saw Bobby Flay make on his show Beating Bobby Flay. I put my own twist on it to make it my own. I use this to toss with salads, dressing for fish and chicken, mix into dips and guacamole to name a few.

Salsa Verde

- 2 cups fresh Cilantro leaves and stems chopped
- 4 tablespoons chopped (diced) onion
- 1 capful Apple Cider Vinegar or Lime Juice
- ¼ cup oil
- Salt and Pepper

Combine all in a glass bowl and mix thoroughly. Leave at room temperature for about 30 minutes before serving. Will keep in the refrigerator, covered, for 3 or 4 days just fine. Store in a glass jar with a tight fitting lid.

I have also put this in my food chopper and turned it into a lovely dressing. Just add equal amount of water to the oil you added and then Italian seasonings AFTER removing from the blender or chopper. Stir well.

Add handfuls of chopped Cilantro to your salads, toss with broasted chicken, fold into mashed cauliflower, sauces and gravies. Also tasty in an omelet.

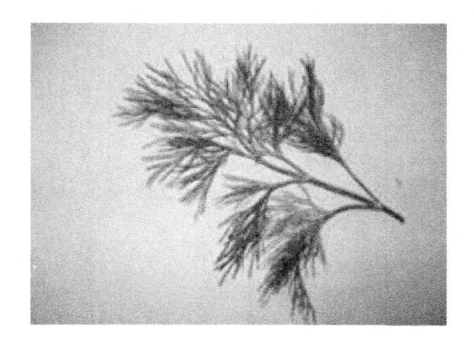

65 DILL

From the celery family, Dill is an annual herb, so great for growing at home. Plant this next to your lettuce but not your carrots. Dill is known to reduce the growth of carrots if grown near them.

According to the onlinelibrary.wiley.com and www.ncbi.nlm.nih.gov/pmc/articles/PMC3249919/

Dill is a good source of:

- Vitamin A
- Vitamin C
- Folate
- Riboflavin

Try adding chopped dill to the pan juices after cooking chicken, add garlic and lemon juice for a nice sauce. Add to homemade dressings and dips! Pairs well with seafood and spinach.

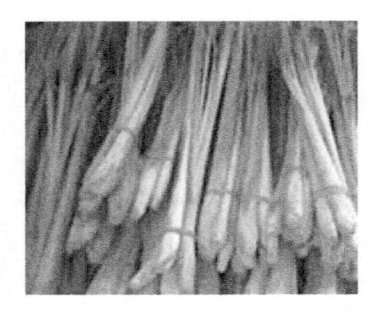

66 LEMONGRASS

Q: What does lemongrass taste like?
A: A light, tangy, lemony flavor. If citrus bothers you, this is a nice substitute for those dishes that call for a squeeze of lemon.

According to spiceography.com Lemongrass is a source of:

- Vitamin A
- Vitamin C
- Folate
- Riboflavin
- Copper
- Zinc
- Magnesium

They go on to suggest that lemongrass could offer the following health benefits:

- Antioxidant
- Antifungal
- Boost immune system
- Diuretic
- Aids in digestion
- Improves problems with constipation as well as diarrhea
- Can have a calming and sedative effect
- Effective in lowering a fever

Commonly used in Thai Food recipes. Try some at home!

Try this Lemongrass Tea:

1 stalk of fresh lemon grass
Raw, unfiltered Honey (optional)
2 cups water

Combine the lemon grass and the water. Bring to a boil. Remove from heat. Cover and allow to steep for about 10 minutes. Pairs nicely with a Green Tea bag. Sweeten to taste if preferred.

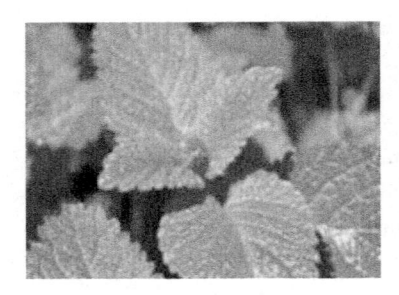

67 MINT

Spearmint or peppermint?

I keep a mint plant in my kitchen. I love smelling the fragrant leaves!

....and when I want a cup of mint tea, or have a recipe that calls for mint its convenient and affordable to just snip off some leaves!

Known to be a calming and soothing herb mint is also said to have antioxidant benefits. According to mercola.com mint also acts as an anti-inflammatory and can alleviate allergy symptoms.

There is a small portion of the population that are bothered by fresh mint in teas, waters and recipes while others find it eases digestive issues and upset stomach. If mint bothers you, simply avoid it.

Nutritional Data on Mint:

- Vitamin A
- Vitamin C
- Iron
- Magnesium

Make a cup of tea by boiling a handful of fresh leaves in a cup of water. Bring to a boil. Remove from heat. Cover. Allow to steep for about 10 minutes. Strain the tea into your cup as to keep out the leaves. Enjoy.

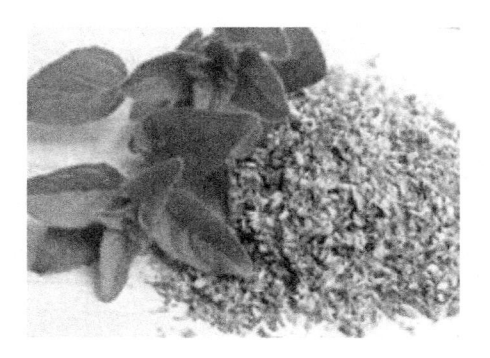

68 OREGANO

From the mint family, oregano is a common staple in most households.

Health benefits of oregano:

- Vitamin K
- Magnesium
- Potassium
- Iron
- Calcium

Known to reduce inflammation (healthline.com), Oregano is also rich in antioxidants, may aid in fighting off bacteria and infection.

Add fresh chopped oregano leaves to salads, as well as in your soups and stews, gravies and sauces. Chopped fresh leaves are the perfect topper to a pizza and to sprinkle on top of grilled meats.

Try placing chopped oregano, oil, and just a hint of apple cider vinegar, salt and pepper in your chopper. Allow to sit for about 10 minutes prior to serving with meats.

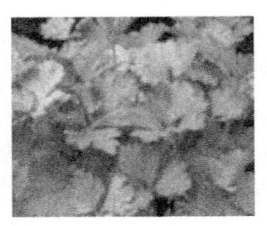

69 PARSLEY

Curly parsley and Flat leaf parsley are the more common varieties found in our local supermarket produce sections. Most find flat leaf parsley to be more versatile and more pleasing to the palate.

A tablespoon of Parsley delivers:

Vitamin A............6%...............RDA
Vitamin C............8%...............RDA
Iron...................1%................RDA
Potassium   21 mg
Vitamin K

Eat more parsley! It's another green leafy. Add it to your salads, sauces and more. Chimichurri is a nice compliment to fish, chicken and roasted vegetables and makes a nice salad dressing too.

- 1 cup fresh parsley
- 2 green onions, chopped
- ¾ cup oil
- 1 tablespoon lime juice
- Salt and pepper

Rustically chop the parsley and onions in your chopper. Then, add oil, lime juice, salt and pepper. Pulse a few more times to blend well. Remove and adjust salt or lime juice to taste. I am sensitive to citrus and find apple cider vinegar works fine as a substitute for the lime juice.

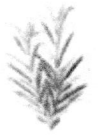

70 ROSEMARY

Rosemary grows wild in some parts of Australia

According to the University of Maryland, umm.edu, Rosemary is used in Europe for indigestion having the approval of the GCE which examines the safety of herbs. They go on to cite a study where 84 people with alopecia (hair loss) massaged their scalps with a Rosemary Oil blend every day for seven months. The study showed those who used the Rosemary Oil blend showed a significant regrowth of hair.

If you take blood thinners like Plavix, Coumadin (warfarin) or a daily aspirin you should know that Rosemary, the herb, may interfere, affecting the body's ability to clot.

Rosemary, used as the fresh woody herb (sometimes chopped or ground) in foods offers:

- Vitamin A
- Thiamin
- Magnesium
- Fiber

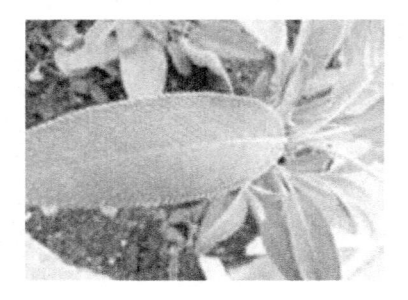

71 SAGE

Mercola has an interesting article on the health benefits of Sage (foodfacts.mercola.com/sage)

In part, the article states that sage, made into a tea, using fresh sage leaves, is known as the "thinkers tea" and has been known to ease depression.

Sage is a source of:

Vitamin K
Vitamin A
Calcium
Potassium
Vitamin C
Vitamin B6
Iron and magnesium

Fresh sage is your best source. If you don't have an outdoor space try container gardening to have this versatile herb at your fingertips!

Sage is most widely used in chicken dishes, add to ground pork for a breakfast sausage taste profile as well as pork chops, creamed onions, Butternut squash soup and more.

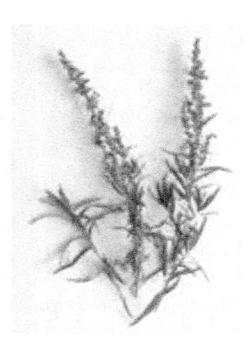

72 TARRAGON

Fresh tarragon has a much more intense flavor then dried. In fact, they hardly resemble the same food. Keep this in mind when using in a recipe.

For those of you who do not like fresh tarragon here are some substitutions:
Fresh basil leaves

Substitutions for dried tarragon: marjoram, oregano, rosemary or dried basil.

An excellent source of :

- Magnesium
- Iron
- Zinc
- Calcium
- Vitamin A
- Vitamin C
- And Tarragon contains antioxidants

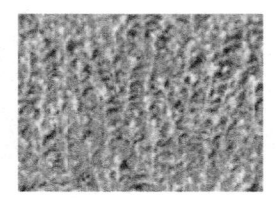

73 THYME

Thyme is a good source of:

- Vitamin K
- Vitamin C
- Fiber
- Riboflavin
- Iron

Thymol is an active ingredient in Thyme. Organicfacts.net states thymol has the ability to aid in the prevention of fungal infections. Thyme is known to be one of the highest sources of antioxidants of any other herb and known to stimulate the production of red blood cells, boosting circulation.

Have you ever made Thyme Tea? Thyme tea can ease menstrual cramps, sooth digestion, aid sleep and boost your immune system. Thyme tea is for the occasional medicinal use and not for consumption as your "every day go-to tea". Too much thyme tea can cause nausea, headaches, and even stomach pains.

Recipe:

1 teaspoon dried thyme leaves
2 cups water
1 teaspoon raw honey
Slice of lemon (optional)

Bring the water to a boil. Turn down to a simmer. Add the dried thyme leaves and cover the pot. Allow to steep for about five (5) minutes. Strain the tea into your cup before drinking.

74 ROOTS AND BULBS

Garlic, ginger, horseradish, and turmeric

All four of these can be found fresh in your produce department and simply place each in their own freezer bag for up to six (6) months. All are gluten free, dairy free, nightshade free and soy free and magnificently healthy!

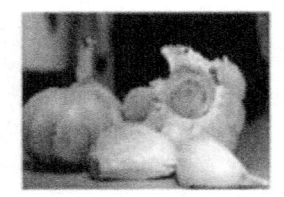

75 GARLIC

Garlic. Not everyone loves garlic but for those of you who do there are great health benefits from using fresh garlic as a part of your regular diet. Remember that you can buy fresh garlic in the produce department and then simply place it in a freezer bag. Just place the entire bulb with the skin on and skin it as you need it or, go ahead and prep the garlic by removing the skin but do not cut the garlic bulbs. Just remove the skins for quick use as needed later.

Health benefits of garlic:

One ounce of garlic delivers:

Manganese................23% RDA
Vitamin B6.................17% RDA
Vitamin C..................15% RDA
Selenium...................06% RDA

There are also trace amounts of copper, potassium, phosphorus and iron.

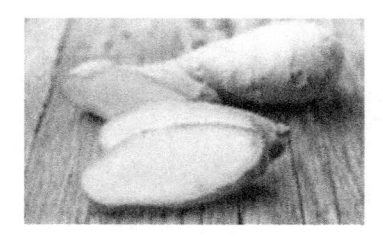

76 GINGER ROOT

Often used to calm an upset stomach, if you find that ginger causes you stomach cramps simply omit this from your diet. Most, but not all people, find ginger to be a comforting food.

Ginger is a wonderful root to keep in the freezer. Simply place the root in a freezer bag. When you need some just grate or cut off just what you need and return the remaining root to the freezer.

Ginger makes a soothing tea for anytime but certainly when you are experiencing nausea or a stomach ache. I also encourage you to look for some recipes using ginger and brighten up your palate!

Ginger offers a good source of:

- Folate
- Vitamin C
- Fiber
- Iron
- Calcium
- Protein
- Niacin
- Riboflavin
- Potassium
- Selenium

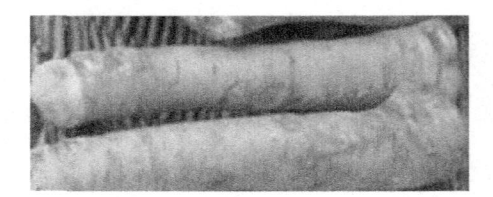

77 HORSERDISH ROOT

Another root vegetable that is easy to purchase in the produce section and simply place in a freezer bag. Please know that it is best to use gloves when handling fresh horseradish root. Much like hot peppers, you do not want to touch your eyes or skin while handling. Be careful! If you can find a jarred horseradish without added unhealthy ingredients that is perfectly acceptable as we generally use very little, it keeps in the refrigerator for quite some time and by itself, horseradish root is gluten free, dairy free, soy free, grain free and it is NOT a nightshade.

A good source of:

- Potassium
- Vitamin C
- Magnesium
- Calcium
- Folate

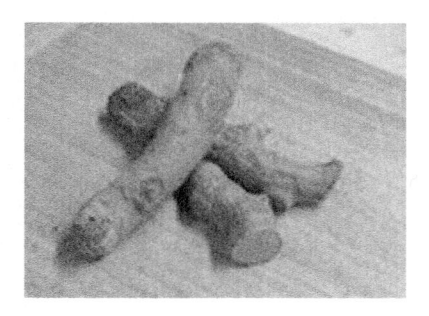

78 TURMERIC

Turmeric has gained popularity in the last few years for its anti-inflammatory properties. If you are sensitive to foods with a high level of potassium you should know that 1 tablespoon of turmeric contains 172 mg of Potassium.

Good source for:

- Potassium
- Fiber
- Calcium
- Vitamin C
- Vitamin B6
- Magnesium

79 HEALTHY FATS

Healthy fats can increase your absorption of fat-soluble vitamins including vitamins A, D, E and K.

Some good sources of healthy fats:

- Avocados
- Black olives
- Egg Yolks
- Flaxseed, ground or milled
- Herring
- Mackerel
- Nuts
- Olive Oil
- Peanut Oil
- Safflower Oil
- Salmon
- Sardines
- Seeds
- Trout
- Tuna

80 HEALTHIEST FOODS BY RANKING

Which foods showed up on our nutrients lists the most?
.....making them the healthiest foods

By far, outweighing any other food, are **dark green leafy vegetables**, like spinach, kale, swiss chard, collard greens, and turnip greens, are so full of nutritious goodness they showed up no less than 40 times on our foods with healthy vitamins, minerals and nutrients.

The next healthiest food, Broccoli, made 16 appearances. Broccoli, a cruciferous vegetable, is known for its many health benefits. For those of you that have been diagnosed with hypothyroidism and perhaps warned to stay away from cruciferous vegetables, many find that simply cooking the vegetables and avoiding raw they do not have any issues to be concerned with. However, if you do find that cruciferous vegetables bother you even when cooked simply eliminate them from your diet. There are plenty of other healthy foods for you to choose from.

How about that incredible edible egg? Coming in third by showing up on 14 lists. Almost all of that nutritional value is coming from the yolk. So, unless your doctor has instructed you to limit your eggs, I would encourage you to look for some egg recipes and enjoy this low carb healthy food.

Food Ranking

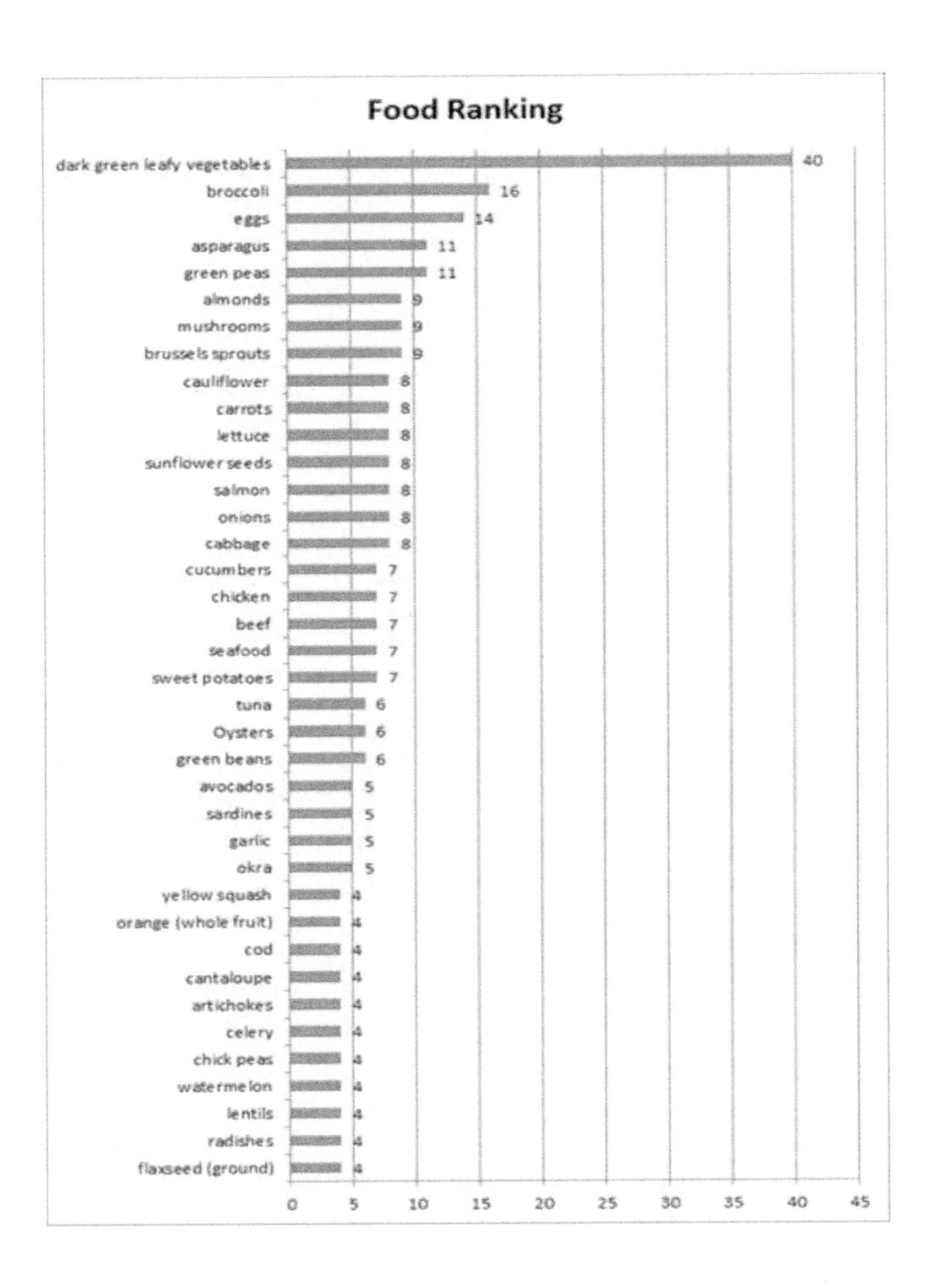

Food	Value
dark green leafy vegetables	40
broccoli	16
eggs	14
asparagus	11
green peas	11
almonds	9
mushrooms	9
brussels sprouts	9
cauliflower	8
carrots	8
lettuce	8
sunflower seeds	8
salmon	8
onions	8
cabbage	8
cucumbers	7
chicken	7
beef	7
seafood	7
sweet potatoes	7
tuna	6
Oysters	6
green beans	6
avocados	5
sardines	5
garlic	5
okra	5
yellow squash	4
orange (whole fruit)	4
cod	4
cantaloupe	4
artichokes	4
celery	4
chick peas	4
watermelon	4
lentils	4
radishes	4
flaxseed (ground)	4

Remember that for optimum health REPLACE your unhealthy foods with healthier choices. If you continue to eat unhealthy foods and ADD healthy foods, as some do, you will be adding more calories into your diet and many find they gain weight. Not to mention that the unhealthy choices will hinder all the good the healthy foods are meant to do for you.

The Ranking List is an excellent place to start.
A nice balance of the food groups!

17 Vegetables
12 Proteins
4 Fruits
4 Other (various)
1 Carbohydrates/starch

81 SUBSTITUTIONS CHART

Many times a substitution is meant as a suitable alternative only and not meant to replace an ingredient to replicate the same exact flavor and texture as before. Much like fruit is suggested as a healthier alternative to cake, brownies or ice cream. The fruit is not going to taste like cakes and ice cream. Likewise, don't expect these foods to taste exactly like the foods they are replacing. My suggestion to my clients is during the first 45 days of transitioning to a healthier diet, choose foods that you already love that are naturally healthy. Focus on those for the time being. The more healthy, unprocessed foods you eat while eliminating processed foods you will find that your taste buds start to change. These healthier substitutions will taste great after your palate has had a chance to be cleansed of 20 plus years of processed foods, and too much sugar, sodium and artificial ingredients.

For example a good alternative to using syrup would be to mash fresh berries with a small amount of raw honey. Warm, and use in place of syrup or jam. To make a more syrup like consistency just put in the blender and puree.

HEALTHY CHOICES, HEALTHY YOU

this   for   that

Food Substitutions

Red Wine	Beef Broth
White Wine	Chicken Broth
Cows Milk	Almond Milk or Broth
Pasta	Spaghetti Squash
Cornstarch	Arrowroot
Raw Tomatoes	Cucumbers, Black Olives
Cooked Tomatoes	Canned Artichokes
Spaghetti Sauce	Pesto, Nomato Sauce
Baked Potato	Baked Sweet Potato
Rice	Diced Yellow Squash
Eggplant	Zucchini
Soy Sauce	Coconut Aminos

Citrus Juice	Zest
Buns	Lettuce Leaves, GF tortillas
Sliced Bread	Lettuce leaves, GF tortillas
Wheat Flour	Almond Flour
Sugar	Raw Honey, Stevia
Mashed Potatoes	Mashed Cauliflower
Bell Pepper	Celery, Radishes
Beer and Vodka	Wine, Tequila, Distilled Liquors
Fat from dairy milk	1 cup water mixed with 1 egg yolk per 1 cup dairy milk (baking)
Paprika	Cumin
Hot Peppers	Onions, Radishes, Black Pepper, Horseradish
BBQ Sauce	Mustard and Honey flavor profiles, Sesame Oil Asian flavors, Nomato
Rice Flour	Tapioca Flour, Almond Flour

82 EXCEPTIONS

Once you have gone through your initial 45 day period of elimination you may have found some foods you can tolerate in limited amounts while still maintaining good health.

Although unprocessed, fresh foods are more favorable to good health, as discussed earlier, there are some processed foods, like cooking oil, nonstick sprays and vinegars that are processed that we use, in small amounts. Here are a few exceptions used in very small limited amounts for cooking and enhancing your healthy choices.

- Bacon: small amounts to enhance vegetables like brussels sprouts for example, or the occasional Pasta Carbonara. Bacon as a side dish should be avoided. The reason is that it is cured: raising the sodium and sugars to an unhealthy level. Lunchmeat should be treated the same as it is cured and lunchmeat is highly processed.
- Parmesan Cheese: used to merely sprinkle on occasion to enhance some foods. I suggest writing the date on your Parmesan Cheese container at the time of your first use. This will help you to not eat it too quickly. Parmesan cheese should only be purchased, if at all, approximately once every 4-6 months.
- Real Butter: while real, unsalted butter may not cause you any unpleasant symptoms it is not as good for you as a healthy oil. If unsalted butter does not taste good to you don't worry. It will taste better as you continue to eliminate overly processed packaged foods.

The more meals you can eat without any exceptions the better your health will be and the better you will feel.

83 CREATE YOUR OWN LIST

A common question from my clients as a nutritionist is how to recreate their favorite dishes that traditionally have foods that are now off limits.

My suggestion to you is to start a list of foods you like that do not require any substitutes or changes. Continue to add to the list; writing them down as they occur to you.

For example:

If you are new to avoiding dairy but love pizza or lasagna with lots of cheese my suggestion is to not try to prepare or eat pizza and/or Lasagna without the cheese and think you are going to like it. It will not be the same. Wait until after your palate has been cleansed of processed foods. Then give it a try with the new ways you have learned to prepare foods. You may also find you can enjoy your favorite foods, once in a while, without changing a thing and without consequence, once your self-discipline has improved.

My suggestion is to avoid dishes you traditionally like that have the foods you are now avoiding or have eliminated. Instead focus on foods you already love that do not have any of the foods you have now eliminated. Make a list of those foods. Start now and add to it as they come to mind. This will help when that moment comes and you "can't think of anything to fix for dinner"!

Do you love Thai foods?   What about roasted chicken?

Pot Roast and vegetables? How about steak? Chicken Piccata? Shrimp Scampi? Do you like spaghetti squash? Roasted vegetables? Onion soup?

Write a few down right now while we are talking about it!

....

....

....

....

84 GO-TO MEAL FAVORITES

We all have those go-to meals; baked chicken, meatloaf, lasagna, macaroni and cheese. Habits we have formed over the last 20 years or so.

Forming new habits can and will happen, but it takes time. It helps, in the beginning, to write these new dishes down so you can reference them at a glance.

This is great for the go-to regular meals (the new healthy ones!) Write them down once you start finding out what they are for you and your family.

As you start to change your diet this can be very helpful for those days that you just can't think of anything to prepare, or use as a reference when planning a trip to the grocery store.

So as you start your journey to healthier meals and as you find out which ones you like and will want to make again write them down here!

Monday

Breakfast
Carrot Puree or Baked Sweet Potato

Lunch
Tossed mixed vegetable salad

Dinner
Poached Chicken and a vegetable

Tuesday

Breakfast
Eggs

Lunch
Pure vegetable soup

Dinner
Meatloaf and vegetables

Wednesday

Breakfast
Melon/Berries

Lunch
Roasted Mixed Vegetables (Baked and hit with the broiler)

Dinner
Seafood and vegetables

Thursday

Breakfast
Avocado Toast

Lunch
Cream of Broccoli Soup

Dinner
Portabella Mushroom and Baked Sweet Potato

Friday

Breakfast
Flaxseed Pancake w/Honey

Lunch
Stir Fry

Dinner
Turkey burger (no bun) with roasted zucchini halves

Saturday

Breakfast
Small apple and half an orange

Lunch
Roasted Romaine Heart with Artichoke and Onion Simmer

Dinner
Baked Chicken on Cream of Asparagus "soup"

Sunday

Breakfast
Frittata

Lunch
Leftover Vegetables

Dinner
Cod fish tacos and cumin stir fried veggies

Notes:

In the Frig: Brussel sprouts, carrots, celery, onions, iceberg, romaine, Sesame Oil, Coconut Aminos, Almond Milk, gluten free tortillas

In the Freezer: peas, chopped spinach/kale, broth, whole okra, garlic, ginger root

Use leftovers if any!

Four (4) Blank meal planners are included in the companion workbook

Monday

Breakfast
Lunch
Dinner

Tuesday

Breakfast
Lunch
Dinner

Wednesday

Breakfast
Lunch
Dinner

Thursday

Breakfast
Lunch
Dinner

Friday

Breakfast
Lunch
Dinner

Saturday

Breakfast
Lunch
Dinner

Sunday

Breakfast
Lunch
Dinner

Notes:

85 BANNED FOODS LIST

One way to start choosing healthier foods is to also start banning the unhealthy foods. One at a time is suggested but whatever you are comfortable with. It is important to master each Banned Food as to build your confidence in your ability to be self-disciplined. We all have self-discipline, but when it comes to food choices many of us "think" we do not.

Start with a food you currently eat; but one you eat seldom. Say donuts. That is the one I started with myself many years ago. I did not buy donuts for consumption at home, but someone would inevitably bring donuts into the office on Fridays where I worked at the time.

I took a sheet of paper and wrote BANNED FOODS at the top and placed it on my refrigerator where I could see it every day. I wrote donuts on the first line. Took a breath and mentally DECIDED that I would no longer eat donuts. Banned for good. Never to be eaten again. A life decision. Donuts had no place in my diet. And with that I faced the next Friday in the office and the donuts. I bravely walked passed them. Watched others eat them. But I honored my decision. I got through the day without eating a donut. It felt good. I felt proud of myself. As each week came and went and the Fridays at the office with the donuts I felt that much more confident in my ability to be self-disciplined. That was 20 years ago and I have never eaten a donut again.

It was about a month after writing DONUT on the BANNED FOODS LIST that I felt confident enough to add another food item. I thought about it for about a week before deciding on pop-tarts. Next it was French fries.

These exercises in self-discipline flooded over into other things. A few years into my BANNED FOODS LIST is when I made the decision to stop smoking once and for all. I finally felt like I could successfully quit and I did. I encourage you to start your own BANNED FOODS LIST.

Some suggestions for your own Banned Foods List

Candy
French fries
Cold cereal
Cookies
Ice cream
Milk shakes
Donuts
Pastry
Anything breaded
Skittles
Brownies
Candy bars
Muffins (even bran)
Cola
Juice
Potato chips
Pretzels
Crackers (all)

86 STAPLES TO HAVE ON HAND

If you are new to transitioning into a healthier diet you may be a bit puzzled about staples to have on hand. I mean how can you have staples in the pantry if everything you are eating is fresh and unprocessed? Right?

While we want to avoid processed foods as much as possible we do need a few of them in order to aid in the preparation of our healthier foods and of course, for some foods, like oil, processed is the only way we can get them into our diet. Presumably support foods will be used sparingly or on rare occasion and will not be the bulk of your food consumption. Here are some general tips when choosing some of your staples:

- Read their labels. Even those foods you have been buying for years. Know what you are eating.
- A canned, jarred or otherwise packaged food with an ingredient label should be limited to 3 ingredients or less. If you pick up something with a long list of you need not worry about all those ingredients that you can't pronounce because as soon as you see those listed you should put it back on the shelf. Those are overly processed foods and not in keeping with your new fresh foods diet.
- The ingredients listed should be available for purchase separately at any supermarket.
- The ingredients should be on your new approved foods lists.

I wanted to give you a SAMPLE LIST OF STAPLES.

My own pantry and staples looks something like this:

FYI: I eat 99% gluten free, dairy free, grain free, soy free and nightshade free. The 1%: You will see some foods listed that I eat only once a month or less, in very small portions.

In the cupboard:

- Apple Cider Vinegar (raw, unfiltered)
- Artichokes, canned or jarred
- Asparagus, canned (great for a quick Cream of Asparagus soup made with chicken broth)
- Arrowroot
- Almond flour
- Baking powder, Baking Soda
- Bisquick Gluten free flour (an exception: see Ch: 82)
- Canned carrots and sliced beets
- Capers
- Coconut oil
- Green beans, canned. No Salt, no soybean oil
- Honey, raw
- Kraut
- Nonstick Cooking Spray: Olive Oil
- Black olives
- Olive oil
- Onions, fresh from produce
- Seasoning and spices (no nightshades)
- Sunflower oil
- Vanilla flavoring or extract
- Water chestnuts

There are of course more and/different foods you can choose to keep as staples in your own kitchen. Just remember the rule of 3 ingredients or less so that you know you are choosing the minimally processed foods with only ingredients you are familiar with.

In the freezer:

- Broccoli
- Broth (homemade; some in 1 cup freezer containers, some from ice cubes)
- Cauliflower
- Cranberries (purchased fresh in produce dept, placed in freezer bag)
- Green peas
- Garlic bulbs (purchased in produce dept; placed in freezer bag)
- Ginger root (purchased in produce department, placed in a freezer bag)
- Kale (chopped)
- Meat and seafood
- Onions: diced and frozen from fresh or frozen Pearl Onions
- Peas and carrots
- Spinach

Staples in the Refrigerator:

- Almond Milk; unflavored original
- Apple, Gala
- Balsamic vinegar
- Butter, real/unsalted
- Carrots
- Celery
- Coconut Aminos
- Cucumbers
- Eggs
- Horseradish
- Lettuce: iceberg and romaine usually
- Mustard
- Olive Oil Mayo
- Parmesan Cheese
- Sesame Oil

Build your own list of staples. Start with foods you already know you like that would qualify: There are ready to pages for your own lists in The Companion Workbook

In the cupboard:

In the freezer:

....

....

....

....

....

....

....

....

In the Refrigerator:

....

....

....

....

....

....

....

....

87 INVENTORY AND MEAL IDEAS

So you went to the grocery store over the weekend and you hid your vegetables in a drawer.

Do you have meals planned around the fresh vegetables you purchased?
If you don't have enough meals planned to be sure you will consume all of the vegetables you bought do that today!

Start by writing down what you purchased in one column. And then your menu ideas in the other. Post that on your refrigerator and cross vegetables off as they have been consumed and are no longer available

Like many others, when I first started eating more produce, I threw out some every week. It would go bad! I have since mastered how much to buy and I have conceded that in order for my produce to NOT-GO-BAD I have to actually eat it!

- Strive to have a fresh component at every meal
- Understand that at first you might get over-zealous and buy too much. Look up recipes and possible ways to freeze your excess.
- Pay attention and learn to buy just what you will eat
- Plan meals around your produce, making sure they are a part of the menu

Every week upon returning from the grocery store I write down what I bought:
- Produce
- frozen foods
- cupboards

I originally started this habit when I was first changing my diet entirely to unprocessed foods. This helped me to remember the produce in the refrigerator, planned for it and made sure it was eaten in an effort to not waste the produce! It also really helps in menu planning.

A sample of what my own Inventory and Menu Ideas looks like:

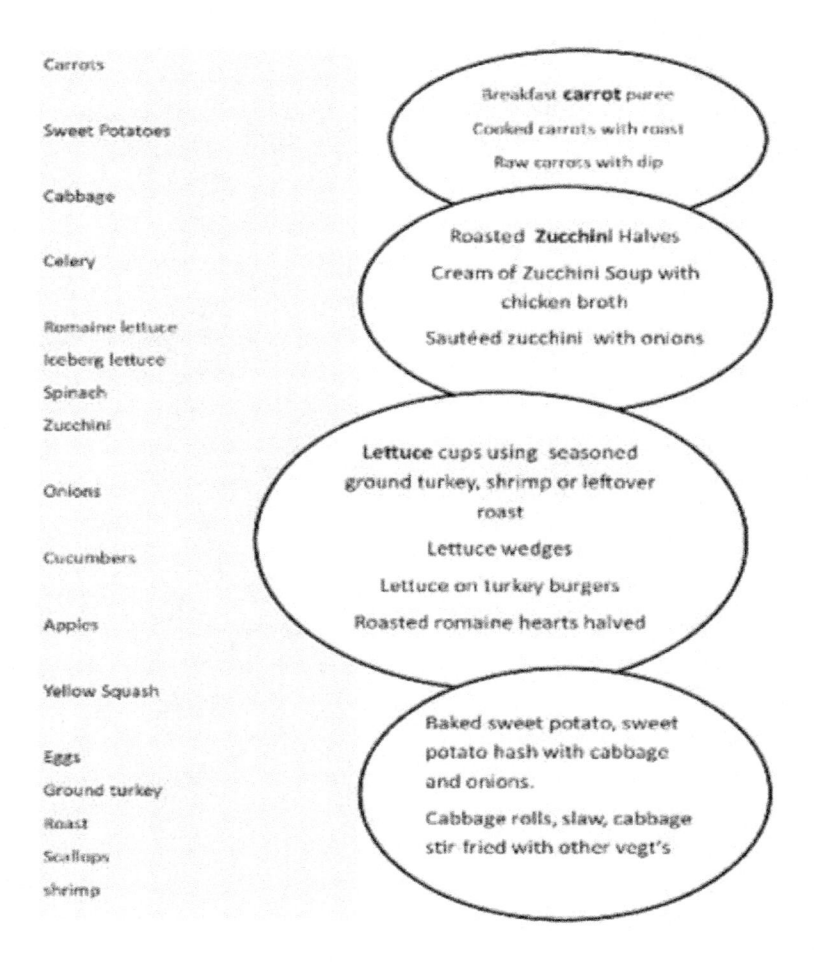

Carrots

Sweet Potatoes

Cabbage

Celery

Romaine lettuce
Iceberg lettuce
Spinach
Zucchini

Onions

Cucumbers

Apples

Yellow Squash

Eggs
Ground turkey
Roast
Scallops
shrimp

- Breakfast **carrot** puree
- Cooked carrots with roast
- Raw carrots with dip

- Roasted **Zucchini** Halves
- Cream of Zucchini Soup with chicken broth
- Sautéed zucchini with onions

- **Lettuce** cups using seasoned ground turkey, shrimp or leftover roast
- Lettuce wedges
- Lettuce on turkey burgers
- Roasted romaine hearts halved

- Baked sweet potato, sweet potato hash with cabbage and onions.
- Cabbage rolls, slaw, cabbage stir fried with other vegt's

Try It Yourself! Write down the fresh produce, meats and seafood you have. Then, using the circles write down how you can use them this week! There are four (4) charts for you to use in The Companion Workbook ISBN 1984237527

HEALTHY CHOICES, HEALTHY YOU

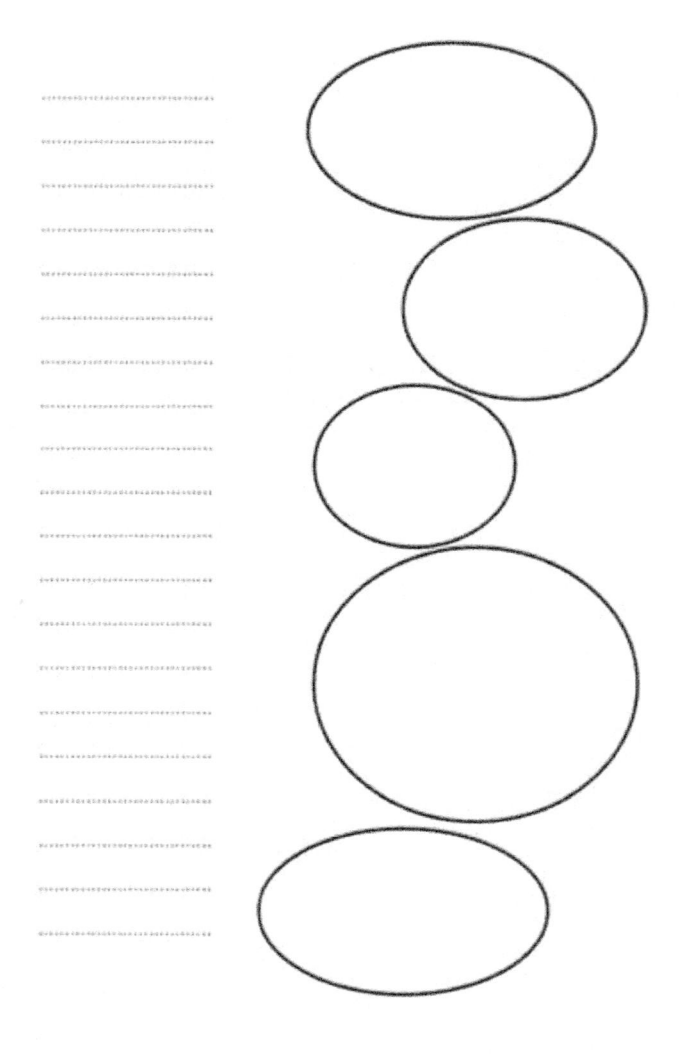

88 NEW FOODS

Once a week or once a month try a new vegetable or seafood. Or, perhaps, revisit a food you tried once long ago and instead, find a new way to prepare it. Much like not liking our Grandmas Brussels sprouts, but we now love them when bought fresh or frozen, cut in half, tossed in oil salt and pepper and baked until tender and golden brown. Also known as roasted brussels sprouts

It is important, and sometimes fun, to try new foods. Make this year the year that you try a new vegetable from the produce department at least once a month. Look up a recipe that looks good to you and your family and you might just find a new food to add to your menu's. You won't like them all, I never have warmed up to the turnip although I do like turnip greens. But I tried it prepared a couple different ways before conceding.

Foods I would like to try:

....

....

....

....

....

....

....

89 DAILY FRESH FOODS

There is nothing like eating fresh foods that have not been cooked. I want to encourage you get into the habit of eating at least one fresh food serving per day. Fresh foods are packed with nutrition as you have learned, and they are very hydrating for the body which is good for your organs, overall health and your skin. They can also be very refreshing after working all day, after a workout, or at a time when you feel stressed or tired.

Here are some suggestions to get you started.

Don't forget that your goal is to eat more vegetables than fruit!

Wedge of Iceberg lettuce. Just pick it up with your hands and eat it like you would a stalk of celery.

Make a fresh food available with every meal; like sliced fresh vegetables or a dip made of fresh vegetables or a Salsa Verde made with fresh herbs.

- Avocado
- Celery
- Radishes
- Carrots
- Cucumbers
- Jicama
- Lettuce (iceberg and romaine)
- Coleslaw (homemade preferably)
- Apple, Pears
- Plum, Nectarine, Orange
- Berries and Melon
- Fresh cut pineapple (not from canned)

Don't get bogged down with traditional breakfast foods either. I find I really like cucumbers at breakfast and guess what? There's nothing wrong with eating cucumbers at breakfast. They are refreshing and bright and a great way to start the day. Romaine lettuce leaves can be eaten with the hand with the vegetable dip like you would a stalk of celery. Layered iceberg leaves make refreshing and tasty hamburger buns and replace taco shells just fine. Don't worry if the rest of your family doesn't eat this way. YOU eat this way. Put it on the table. Be a good example. But always make it available. No one else can CHOOSE to eat fresh vegetables if they aren't even on the table.

90 BEVERAGES

Your best choice of any beverage is water. Plain, clean water.

When I first started my journey to an unprocessed diet I kept reading where we should just drink water and nothing else. Not something I ever thought I would be able to do. Now, it is my go-to beverage. I will occasionally have tea or coffee and on rare occasion wine or cola, but I find I prefer the water. This did not happen overnight. But the more I embraced eating unprocessed foods the more I just wanted water and the other beverages just did not have the same appeal. This will happen for you too.

Beverage that are acceptable on an unprocessed foods diet:

- Almond Milk: unflavored, original
- Coconut water: but please read the label
- Coffee
- Sparkling water: unflavored. Read the label.
- Tea from loose tea leaves or tea bags (not instant tea)
- Water

91 START WHERE YOU ARE

If you have been dancing around a totally unprocessed healthy diet for some time and are ready to go all out then go for it. But if the majority of your food intake is processed, microwavable foods or fast foods then it's okay to start there. Start where you are. One step leads to another. One good choice leads to another. Start by requiring a little of yourself and slowly build your confidence and desire to continue. Use the Banned Foods List to help you get started. If you currently don't buy and eat any foods from the produce department start with one vegetable per week. Something you know you like and commit to eat it that week. Write it down so you know you PLAN on eating it for lunch, or incorporating it into your evening meal. Decide you will start eating a larger portion of vegetables than meat. Small changes matter a lot!

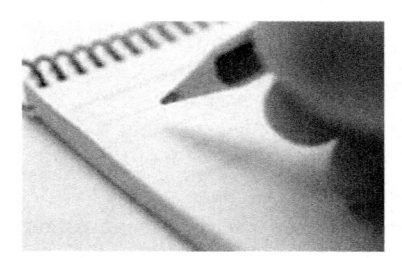

Here are some questions I like to ask each of my clients when I first meet with them. It is important to physically write down your answers. Writing things down will help to impend the idea into the brain and change your thoughts from ideas into action. Answering the following questions now, before beginning is very important. In one year look back at your answers and see how you have improved! Take your time with your answers. If you aren't sure of an answer right now come back in a week and try again.

HEALTHY CHOICES, HEALTHY YOU

1. What is your goal here? To lose weight, eat healthier, or both?

2. Are you at a healthy weight right now? What do you weigh?

3. What weight would you like to be if you feel you need to lose weight?

4. Have you been diagnosed with some health conditions that are made worse by your diet? What are your health issues and symptoms?

5. What foods do you think contribute to your symptoms worsening?

6. Which of these foods do you feel you can stop eating? Perhaps add to the Banned Foods List mentioned in an earlier chapter....

7. Will you still want to eat healthier next year at this time?

8. What are some healthy foods (that you like) you think you SHOULD be eating that you currently do not? Try to name at least 3 healthy foods that would be healthier choices:

9. Why don't you currently eat these foods?

10. What do you think are some things you can do to prioritize your transition to a healthy foods diet? (i.e.: eat at home more often; less at restaurants, take your own lunch, learn how to prepare healthy foods in a quick and timely manner, spend some time looking at recipes for vegetables)

11. Are you open to trying some new foods or learning to prepare fresh foods in a different way?

12. Do you feel a higher grocery bill has been stopping you from eating healthier?

13. If yes, are you willing to use the same amount of grocery budget on fresh foods INSTEAD of processed foods?

14. Do you currently exercise?

15. Do you think exercising more would help you to a healthier body?

16. What types of exercises have you thought about incorporating? Try to name at least 3 different ways to be more active on a regular basis:

I have a list of suggestions for a more active lifestyle in Chapter 1 (included in The Companion Workbook too)

92 WHEN YOU CHEAT

Here is an example of how my calendar looks. I don't write down everything I eat. Instead I write down just when I "cheat" or have foods that I can only tolerate on occasion. This helps me to ensure not eating these foods too often and triggering symptoms or gaining weight. I keep it posted on the refrigerator so I can see it at a glance.

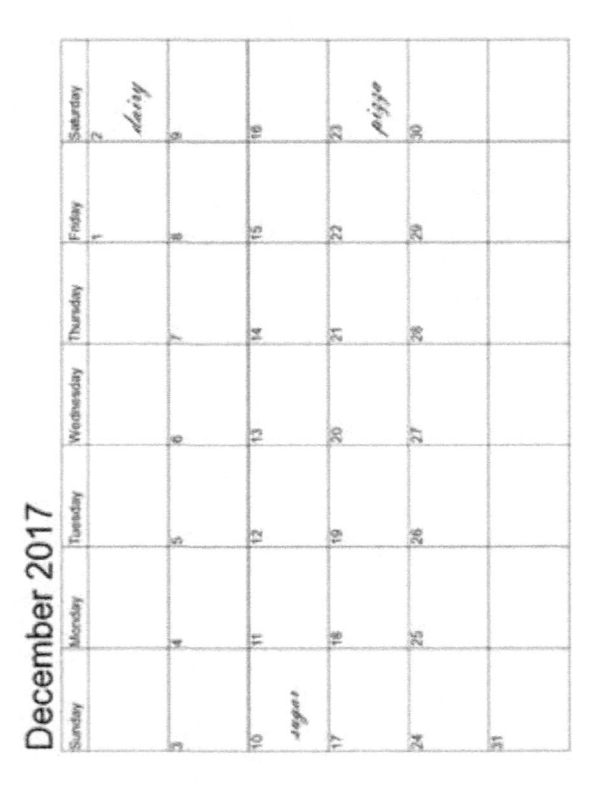

	December 2017					
Sunday	Monday	Tuesday	Wednesday	Thursday	Friday	Saturday
					1	2 *dairy*
3	4	5	6	7	8	9
10	11	12	13	14	15	16
17 *sugar*	18	19	20	21	22	23 *pizza*
24	25	26	27	28	29	30
31						

93 HEALTHY KITCHEN HABITS

- Use Glass, not plastic when storing foods in the refrigerator. Save those pickle, horseradish, and artichoke jars and remove the labels.
- Cool broth to room temperature, uncovered, before refrigerating or freezing. This helps to ward off the possibility of bacteria forming.
- Wash even organic produce. Airborne pathogens and people sneezing during packing are just a few reasons you should always wash fresh produce before consuming.
- Wait to wash all produce until just prior to eating. Fruits, like apples, should be dried off before eating, wiping away any pesticides left behind.
- Don't wash produce until you are ready to eat it. Dry produce last much longer. Keep in an airtight container or Ziploc bag
- Use different designated cutting boards for seafood, chicken and vegetables
- Thaw foods in the refrigerator, not on the counter or sink
- For juicier chicken cover in water while thawing
- Keep nuts and seeds in the refrigerator for up to six months and in the freezer if keeping for up to one year
- Save glass spice jars and buy some labels for your own homemade spice blends
- With just a little bit of planning, healthy food can be your new fast food
- You do not need to add flour, crackers, or even eggs to your meatloaf! This just adds calories you don't need and it's a waste of food. The trick to keeping your meatloaf in a nice, sliceable loaf without fillers is to use lean ground meat, at least 85% lean or higher and use ground meat that has never been frozen. Don't add any liquids; just seasoning
- Store oil in a dark, cool cupboard. Not next to the stove on the counter.
- Store ground flaxseed in the freezer between uses.
- Your refrigerator should be kept at 40 degrees Fahrenheit or below. If your refrigerator does not have a thermometer buy an inexpensive appliance thermometer to set inside.
- Your freezer should be kept at zero or below.

- Melons can be stored on the counter until they have been cut. Store cut melons in the refrigerator.
- Honey, even raw unfiltered honey, should be stored at room temperature and not in the refrigerator. It is normal for raw, unfiltered honey to show some signs of crystallization after a time.

- Store coffee in an air tight container in a cool dark cupboard much like your oil. Not the refrigerator.
- Store uncut onions in dark, cool cupboard at room temperature. Once cut, store inside an air tight container in the refrigerator
- Apples do fine for a week or so on the counter but will last longer when kept in the refrigerator.
- Wash your hands before preparing foods.
- Use glass and stainless steel whenever possible.

According to health.state.mn.us/foodsafety/cook/cooktemp.html
on safe cooking temperatures:

145F = 62C | 160F = 71C | 165F = 74C

- Chicken should be cooked to a minimum of 165 degrees F.
- Pork should be cooked to a minimum 160F
- Ground meat 160 degrees F
- Fish and shellfish 145F
- Beef: whole cuts: rare: 145F, medium: 160F and well done: 170F

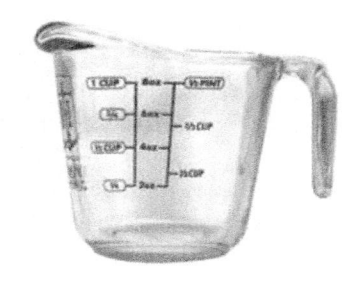

½ cup   =   8 Tablespoons

1 cup   =   8 ounces   =   240 milliliters (mL)

3 teaspoons   =   1 Tablespoon

4 Tablespoons =   ¼ cup

2 cups   =   1 pint

To figure Celsius and Fahrenheit temperatures:

(Celsius degree) X 1.8 + 32 = your Fahrenheit temperature

likewise

(Fahrenheit degree) X 1.8 = your Celsius temperature

Grams to cups conversions depends on the density of the food products you are measuring.

94 HOW THE COUNTDOWN JOURNAL CAN HELP YOU

Use the 60 or 45 Day Countdown method on your wall calendar, or use a Countdown Journal for an elimination period if you are cleansing yourself of glutens, dairy, soy, nightshades, sugars or grains.

The Countdown Method is just as helpful to cleanse your palate and body of processed foods and get your sweet tooth under control and get you on your way to eating a fresh food (unprocessed) diet.

Processed foods, over time, dull the palate. After a palate cleanse (45-60 consecutive days without processed foods) the majority of people find their sweet tooth is tamed, vegetables taste better, and almost all find they no longer crave the carbs they once did. This will go a long way toward making a transition to fresh foods much more enjoyable. The Companion Workbook, ISBN: 1984237527, includes a 45 Day Countdown Journal.

95 CLOSING THOUGHTS

As you finish this book I am hoping you feel ready to embrace fresh foods that will give you a healthier body and that you can begin to think of a life without overly processed foods. As someone who has been through this myself and who has also counseled hundreds of clients I wanted to address some of the most common concerns and anxieties:

Concern over feeling hunger?

Stop eating as soon as you feel full..... You should also eat if you feel hungry.

You should never feel concerned at being hungry when eating healthy. There are lots of low carb foods as well as foods with no carbs. You should eat if you feel hungry, just make better choices. Many of these foods can be made into "comfort" foods like a gravy, creamy sauce, and dips.

You should also know that most people find that once they have eliminated all the processed foods and excess sugar they have no need for snacking between meals and actually feel full on much less food then they would have guessed. I too found this to be true. I eat half what I did during meal times and do not feel the need to snack at all where before my diet changes I was an avid snacker.

Processed foods and sugars cause faux hunger pangs. A person really does *feel* hungry, but may not be. This is the addictive part. Just like nicotine. Having a cigarette is what makes you want another cigarette in an hour or so. Same with processed foods and sugars. Consuming a heavily processed foods diet will only make you crave more food in a few hours. By removing these foods from your diet you won't feel full but neither will you feel hungry. You will just be satisfied. There is the occasion my stomach will growl and I know that somewhere, somehow, over the last 24 hours I have eaten something processed.

Learning when to stop eating is a big part of maintaining a healthy weight and keeping digestive issues at bay. Here are some tips. In the beginning, try this on the weekend or at your evening meal when you are not rushed.

1. Put your food or your utensils down between each bite.
2. Take the time to chew each bite thoroughly before swallowing
3. Count to 10 after swallowing before slowly taking another bite.
4. Repeat.

- When half your food is gone – **stop eating**.
- Wait 5 full minutes. If you are still hungry proceed to eat half of what is left following steps 1-4.

- As soon as you do not feel hungry any longer you should stop eating all together. If you eat until you feel full you have overeaten. It takes your brain about 10-20 minutes to realize you have had enough to eat. Meaning that when you feel full you were most likely full 10-20 minutes ago and everything you ate after that time was food you did not need.

- I recommend an article on this I found at: healthyeating.sfgate.com/stomach-full-stop-eating-3080.html but it is commonly known that our brains take a while to catch up!

- Don't feel obligated to eat the last bite or two. If you aren't hungry anymore stop eating no matter what is still on your plate. Take this as a learning experience and next time put less food on your plate.

Sometimes I just can't think of anything to eat:

Even with a plan we can sometimes just feel at a loss as to what we should eat to stay on our diet. First of all make sure you use some of the worksheets and lists I sample and provide in this book.

Here are some tips:

Remember that for 20 plus years you have created a habit of eating a certain way, eating certain foods. It will take some time for your brain to think of the new, healthier foods as your go-to foods. Be patient. It will happen.

In the meantime, as you transition your way into healthier choices, use the worksheets and charts and write down new healthy favorites that you know you want to make again.

Your quick go-to guide, albeit not exactly exact but great in a pinch, is to remember this:

Fruit for breakfast (fresh fruit only, minimal limited portions and remember eggs are a no-carb food and although not fruit, an excellent choice for breakfast)

Vegetables for lunch: just vegetables! Broth and oils as support foods for preparation are okay but steer clear of meat (for most of us). If you find you get sleepy after your lunch try sticking to just vegetables. The exception here are people who are very labor intense throughout the day and some of those do find they need some meat or seafood with their lunch. Refer to the Protein chapter for a list of vegetables to get your protein if you want to omit the meat. Potatoes and legumes are not vegetables and should be avoided.

Protein for supper: A protein with more vegetables of course! The majority of your meal should still be vegetables when including meat, seafood or other protein. Not the other way around.

Can I transition into eating less processed foods by replacing them a little at a time with fresh foods or should I do it cold turkey?

We are each unique in what works for us. This is up to you and either way is okay.

You've eaten what was supposed to be an approved food and now you feel terrible:

Before you dismiss a food a fresh food, consider how you ate it. Sometimes it isn't *what* we eat but *how* and when we eat it. I mention this because some people are perplexed why a drink of water or a bit of salad or eggs can trigger acid reflux. Sometimes it isn't necessarily the food. If you know you made a good food choice there are other things you should consider:

Did you chew each bite well before swallowing?

Did you overeat? Were you full?

Did you eat when you were not hungry?

What have you eaten in the last 12 hours?

Did you eat too quickly or gulp down a large amount of water all at once?

Why are so many so sick? It seems over the last 20 years we have seen a definite upswing in the number of people who have developed stomach issues, digestive issues, conditions associated with pain not only in the joints and muscles but sometimes all over, not to mention the number of people with diabetes, high blood pressure, sensitivities to dairy, gluten, allergies, and not to mention excess weight and those considered obese. These are just a few health issues that have been on the rise for so many people. We have to ask ourselves why. Why do an alarming number of people have these complaints more than ever before? In the last 30 years diets in the United States have changed drastically.

Fast foods, microwavable pre-cooked dinners, overly processed foods being the majority of what is consumed are often blamed and for sure they are adding to the problem.

I also want to point out some other diet changes often overlooked. I don't know that these changes are the root cause of our health problems today but I do think our eating habits, and how we cook and prepare our foods should be examined.

While I don't believe a poor diet is causing all diseases and conditions I think the lack of nutrition leaves us more vulnerable to disease. Just something to consider.

In the last 20-30 years we have stopped cooking meat on the bone. If you are over 50 like I am you remember your mother cooking a roast with the bone-in. Chicken too always had a bone-in while cooking.

Very few foods were cooked or even warmed in the microwave.

More people had vegetable gardens which has been on the decline with more and more people leaving rural areas for employment and as home prices rise, more apartment and condo dwelling.

Convenience foods are out of control as is the bottled water.

We stopped eating the yolk of the egg opting for just the whites. There are important nutrients in the yolk and it is suggested the whites may be responsible, in part, for some allergies.

Going to a restaurant use to be the occasional treat to celebrate a special event. Many people now stop at a drive through every day for at least one, if not more than one meal a day.

96 RECIPES

Ground Flaxseed Low Carb Pancake Recipe

- 3 tbsp. Flaxseed Meal
- Baking Soda, .25 tsp
- 1/2 teaspoon baking powder
- 1 Egg
- Olive Oil, 1 tsp.
- 1 tablespoon honey
- pinch of salt

Mix well. Cook as you would any pancake but do not flip too soon. Be sure it is showing signs of browning along the edges before turning over. Flip just once for best results. Suggestions: you can, of course, add cinnamon, vanilla, and nutmeg for added flavor. Or try adding pecans! Serve with berries and Raw Honey.

(skinned, poached apricots are delicious with the Flaxseed Pancakes)

I have used this basic recipe, adding a couple tablespoons of water to thin it out and made a nice crepe with fresh fruit. Similarly you could make a cream of chicken with shredded chicken and a dairy free alfredo sauce. Wrap the seasoned chicken with the very thin crepes and cover with your sauce.

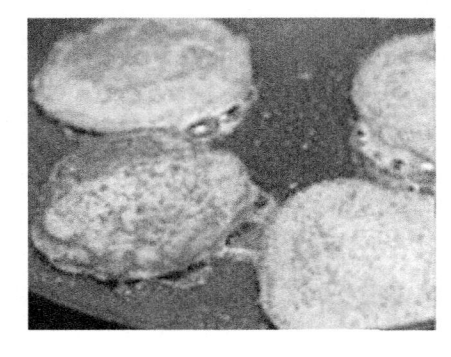

Hydrating Cucumber Vegetable Dip Recipe

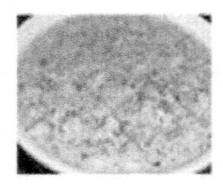

This is a very hydrating and fresh dip that can also be used on sandwiches in place of mayo. This is Very low carb, dairy free, gluten free, nightshade free, soy free and grain free. It is also all fresh and very healthy.
- 1 peeled cucumber, chopped
- ½ cup chopped iceberg lettuce
- 4 tablespoons Sunflower Oil
- 4 tablespoons water
- A pinch of salt and a pinch of black pepper
- 1 capful of Raw, Unfiltered Apple Cider Vinegar

Optional additions to the blender for a different flavor and texture profile:
- 1/8 cup chopped parsley or cilantro
- One drained can of artichokes

Place oil, vinegar, and water in your chopper or blender first. Then add the remaining ingredients. Blend to the consistency you like. Some prefer a more rustic chunky dip while sometimes, like if making a sandwich spread, you may prefer a smoother dip. If you find it is too thin add more lettuce.

Once removed and placed in a bowl, adjust seasonings and vinegar/oil as needed and stir well.

The addition of other seasonings is optional. It is recommended that these seasonings be added after removing from the blender as sometimes it can turn them bitter.

Some suggestions: Italian Seasoning, onion powder, Garlic Powder

Salsa Verde

- 2 cups fresh Cilantro leaves and stems chopped
- 4 tablespoons chopped (diced) onion
- 1 capful Apple Cider Vinegar or Lime Juice
- ¼ cup oil
- Salt and Pepper

Combine all in a glass bowl and mix thoroughly. Leave at room temperature for about 30 minutes before serving. Will keep in the refrigerator, covered, for 3 or 4 days just fine. Store in a glass jar with a tight fitting lid.

I have also put this in my food chopper and turned it into a lovely dressing. Just add equal amount of water to the oil you added and then Italian seasonings AFTER removing from the blender or chopper. Stir well.

Have you ever made Thyme Tea?

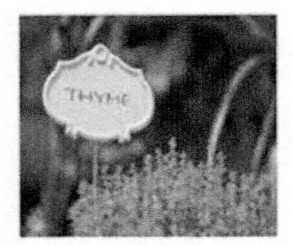

Thyme tea can ease menstrual cramps, sooth digestion, aid sleep and boost your immune system. Thyme tea is for the occasional medicinal use and not for consumption as your "every day go-to tea". Too much thyme tea can cause nausea, headaches, and even stomach pains.

Recipe:

1 teaspoon dried thyme leaves
2 cups water
1 teaspoon raw honey
Slice of lemon (optional)

Bring the water to a boil. Turn down to a simmer. Add the dried thyme leaves and cover the pot. Allow to steep for about five (5) minutes. Strain the tea into your cup before drinking.

Poached Chicken

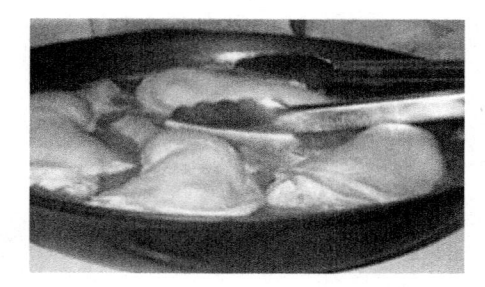

Poaching chicken breasts is a simple and delicious way to enjoy poultry.

Rub your chicken breast "with the rib" (bone-in), with oil, salt and pepper.

Brown on both sides in a hot skillet turning only once.
Wait until the first side is a nice golden brown before turning over. Even if you are using skinless breasts. (this can also be done with bone-in chicken thighs of course). Once both sides are browned remove temporarily from the skillet.

Add just a small amount of water and scrape the bottom of the skillet to loosen up any renderings.

Return the chicken to the skillet and add more water until the chicken is halfway covered. The top of the chicken should not be covered in water.

Bring to a simmer and cover with a lid. Set your timer for 10-20 minutes depending on the size of your chicken pieces.

Try this simple method first to see how you like the basic poached chicken. Then, the next time remember you can always add different seasonings for a different taste profile. Some suggestions would be to add cumin when adding the salt and pepper, or perhaps Italian seasoning. You could also add garlic and/or onions to the water while simmering.

Poached chicken is a great way to prepare chicken that you will shred with a fork or your hands for enchiladas or creamed chicken or to add to soups. Also nice to keep in the refrigerator for sandwiches or lettuce cups.

Dairy Free Cream of Mushroom Soup

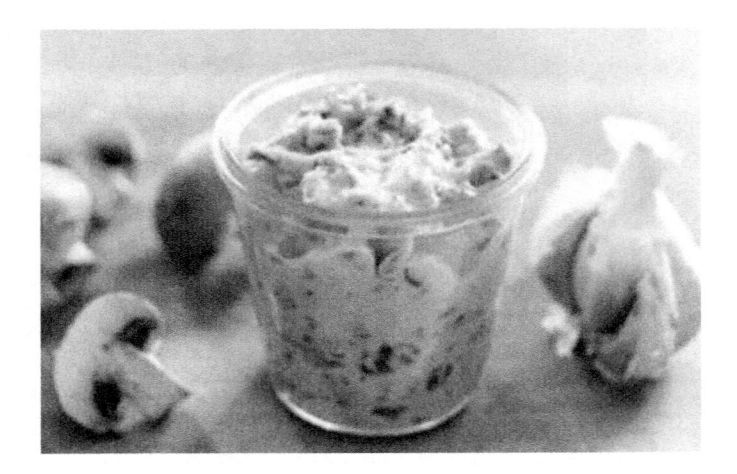

Ingredients:
- ¼ c. real butter
- 1 cup diced fresh mushrooms
- ¼ c. diced yellow onion
- 2 diced garlic cloves
- 4 Tablespoons Arrowroot or Gluten Free flour
- ½ c. Chicken broth

Melt butter in a skillet and add mushrooms and onion. Sauté until tender; about 3-4 minutes. Add garlic and stir. Sprinkle with Arrowroot. Stir to coat. Add broth, a little at a time, stirring as you add it using a fork or whisk.. This should thicken quite quickly. Stop adding chicken stock when the consistency is that of Cream of Mushroom Soup you find in the can. This can be stored in a glass jar and used within the week for Mushroom Soup (add a cup or so more chicken broth) add some carrot if making a soup.

Or, use in Green Bean Casserole as you would store bought Cream of Mushroom Soup, a sauce for steak, pork chops or chicken.

SAGE SAUCE ROASTED CHICKEN

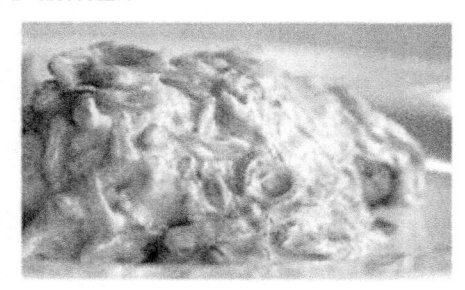

- 4 Chicken breasts or thighs
- Salt and pepper
- 2 tablespoons oil
- 1 leek, chopped
- ¾ cup chicken broth
- ¼ cup dry white wine or dry vermouth
- 2 tablespoons fresh sage leaves (+)
- 2 tablespoons unsalted real butter
- 2 teaspoons Dijon mustard

Preheat oven to 375 degrees.

Salt and pepper the chicken and brown, in oil, both sides, turning just once. In skillet. Transfer chicken to 375 oven. Bake about 15 minutes.

After chicken has baked about 15 minutes add the chopped leeks and ¼ cup of the broth to the skillet with the chicken and continue to bake for another 15 minutes.

When the chicken is done..., set the chicken aside on a platter to rest. Pour the broth and leeks to a skillet on the stove top:

Add remaining broth and the wine. Simmer about 5 minutes to cook out the alcohol. Turn off the heat. Immediately add sage leaves, butter, and mustard to the skillet and stir gently until blended.

Spoon sauce over chicken to serve.

This is one of the recipes from my book: 52 Chicken Recipes and as with all my own published cookbooks and the Grocery List is: #glutenfree #dairyfree #soyfree #lowcarb #nightshadefree and #grainfree A diet that is anti-inflammatory which is known to be very helpful for easing symptoms for those living with an autoimmune issue like arthritis, thyroid, and others.

Roasted Whole Okra

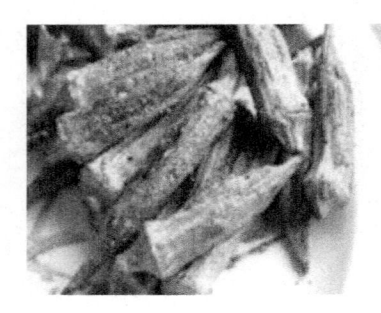

....or zucchini, brussels sprouts, onions, and more!

Preheat your oven to 450 degrees F.

Place whole okra, you can use fresh or frozen, in a glass bowl. Toss evenly with oil, salt and pepper.

Spread evenly onto a baking sheet.

Bake in preheated oven for about 15 minutes or until tender and golden brown as though it is starting to char on the edges. Turn on the broiler if you need to for browning before removing from the oven.

For zucchini, cut fresh only zucchini in half lengthwise. Repeat same steps as above with oil, salt and pepper and baking.

A few seasoning blends that you can make ahead that do not include nightshades or gluten. Make enough for at least half a glass spice jar you have saved and changed the label.

Avoiding cured meats is a great choice when choosing a healthy unprocessed diet. Buy ground pork and add the following seasoning blends prior to cooking:

Breakfast Sausage: sage, oregano, cumin, salt, pepper, garlic. Start with one teaspoon of each except the salt. Add salt a pinch at a time after combining, smelling and tasting all the other seasonings.

Italian Sausage: Italian Seasoning blend from the store with garlic powder, black pepper and salt to taste if needed.

Make meatballs, patties or loose meat and freeze ahead too.

Make meatloaf and freeze ahead too: my meatloaf is simple: ground beef that is at least 83% lean and has never been frozen. Combine with salt, black pepper, garlic powder, and thyme. Form and bake as usual. No need for fillers or extra ingredients. Let people at the table add ketchup if they want or make a mushroom gravy!

For more gluten and dairy free recipes checkout my Amazon Authors page:

http://www.amazon.com/author/paulachenderson

97 BONUS COLORING AND WORD FIND PUZZLE

N	U	T	R	I	E	N	T	S
F	C	H	S	E	R	F	N	E
S	O	O	T	H	Y	I	M	L
E	F	O	D	E	M	P	I	B
P	C	I	D	A	L	L	N	A
I	H	O	T	L	E	A	E	T
C	I	I	R	T	A	N	R	E
E	V	L	D	H	F	T	A	G
R	E	C	A	Y	Y	S	L	E
I	N	N	I	H	C	U	Z	V

VEGETABLES NUTRIENTS ZUCHINNI VITAMINS
MINERAL HEALTHY RECIPES FRESH
FOOD FIT PLANTS LEAFY COD CHIVE
OIL RDA

This and the coloring pages are available in The Companion Workbook (paperback) isbn: 1984237527

HEALTHY CHOICES, HEALTHY YOU

fresh
fit food
HEALTH nutrients
nourish ACTIVE
LIFESTYLE
produce
vitamins
VEGETABLES
LEAFY GREENS

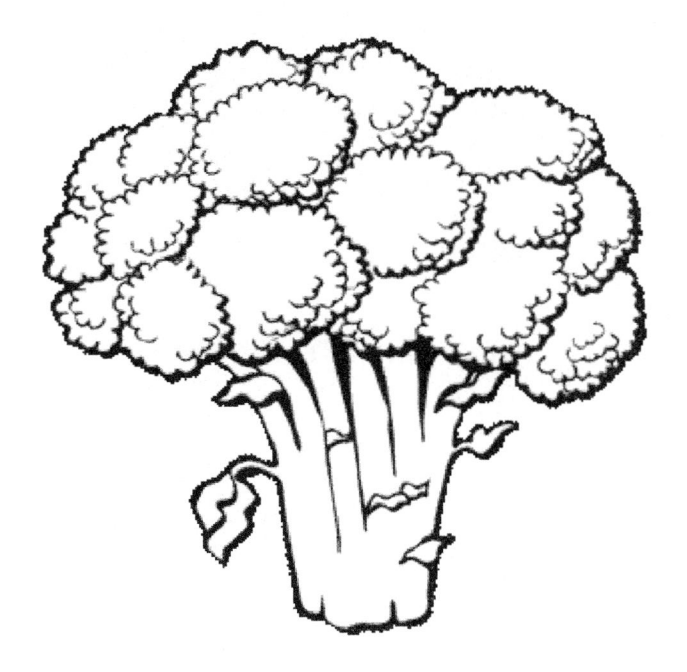

HEALTHY CHOICES, HEALTHY YOU

....

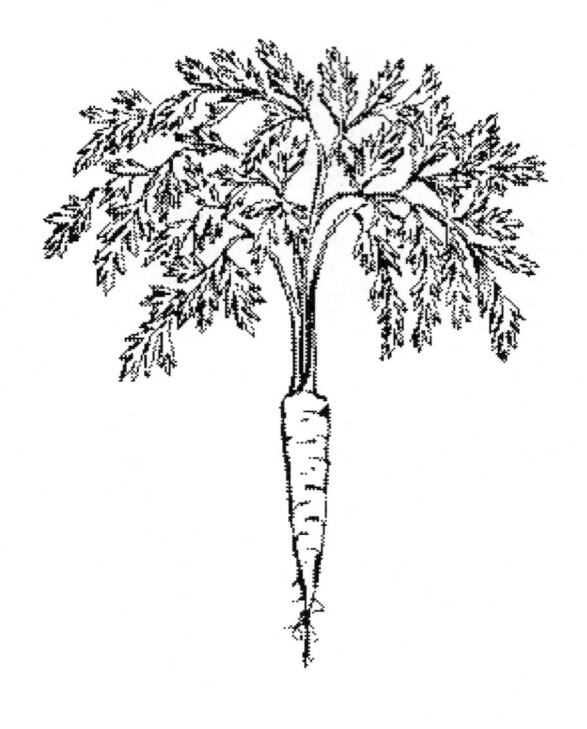

HEALTHY CHOICES, HEALTHY YOU

....

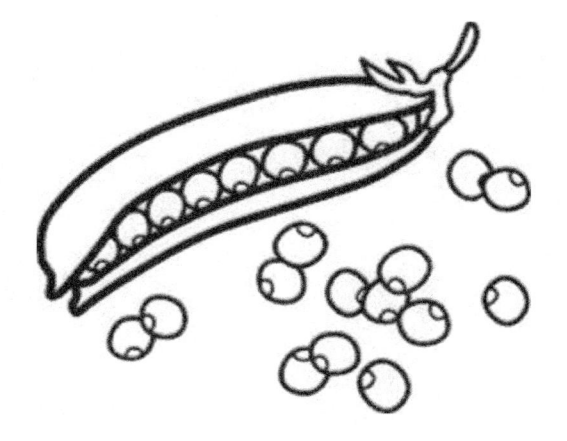

HEALTHY CHOICES, HEALTHY YOU

....

....

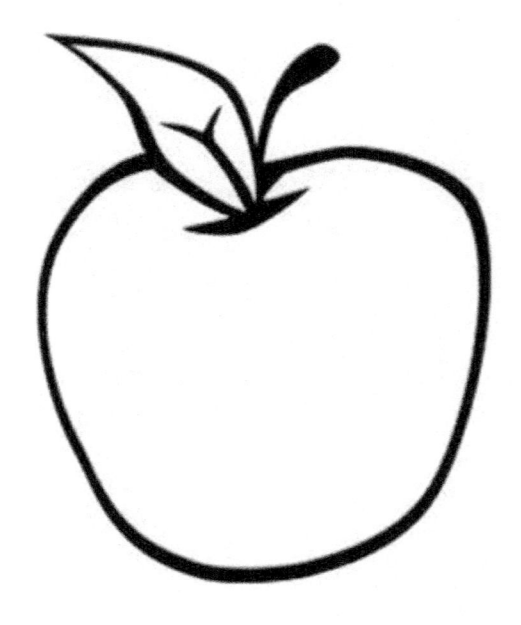

HEALTHY CHOICES, HEALTHY YOU

……..   ……..   ……..   ……..   ……..

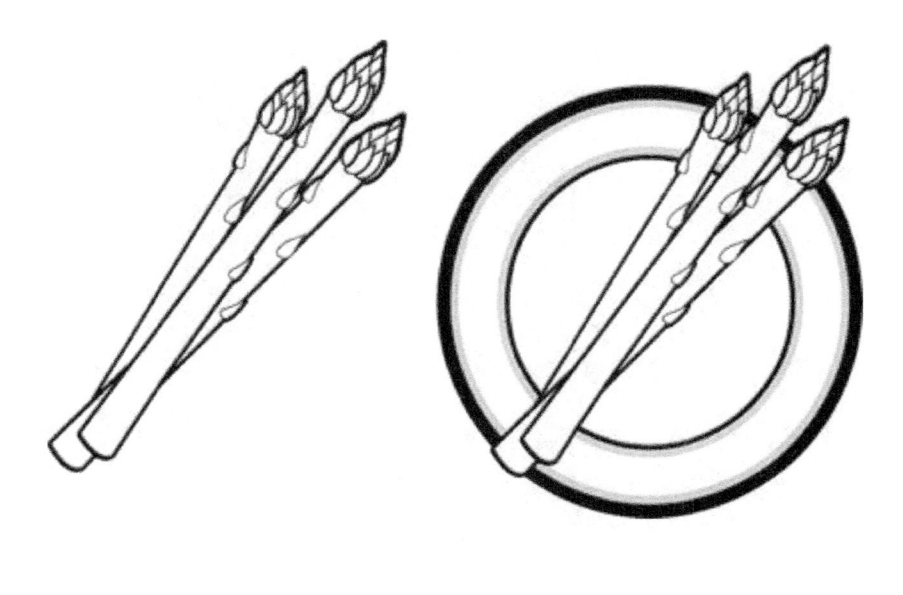

HEALTHY CHOICES, HEALTHY YOU

....

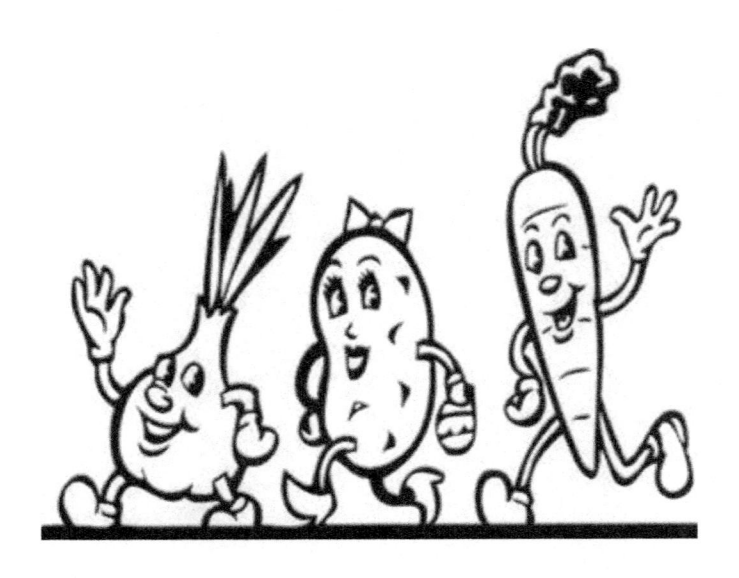

HEALTHY CHOICES, HEALTHY YOU

98 REFERENCES AND SOURCES

Sources for the nutritional data contained in this book are from the following sites. If you are interested in further reading these sites are highly recommended.

The Dietary Reference Intakes (DRIs) was developed by the Food and Nutrition Board (FNB) at the Institute of Medicine (IOM) of the National Academies (formerly National Academy of Sciences)

onlinelibrary.wiley.com
Healthline.com
Mayoclinic.org
Whfoods.com
nutritiondata.self.com
livestrong.com
cdc.gov
womenshealth.gov
lpi.oregonstate.edu/
healthsupplementsnutritionalguide.com
jn.nutrition.org
twofoods.com
ajcn.nutrition.org
arthritis.org

In conclusion:

I want you to crave

what your body needs.

"Not what it has become addicted to"

99 ABOUT THE AUTHOR

Paula C. Henderson makes her home in Las Vegas, Nevada. In 1995 she became a certified weight loss counselor while living in Ohio. This began a passion for sharing the benefits of healthy eating and a healthier lifestyle in general.

An independent publisher, Paula's books can be found in kindle and paperback editions on Amazon.

http://www.amazon.com/author/paulachenderson

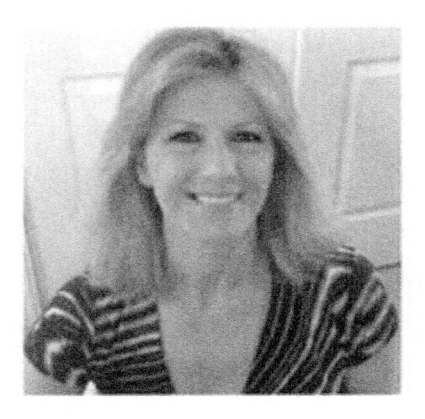

other published works by
paula c. henderson

A Gluten and Dairy Free, Grain Free, Soy Free, and Nightshade Free **Grocery List** http://amzn.to/2CcNSDO

52 Low Carb Healthy! Tasty! **Chicken Recipes**: Gluten Free Dairy Free Soy Free Nightshade Free Grain Free Unprocessed, Low Carb, Healthy Ingredients http://amzn.to/2Cdq6HV

Lettuce Amaze You: 100% Dairy, Gluten, Soy, Nightshade and Grain Free Lettuce Recipes http://amzn.to/2EDbumu

Authors page on amazon:
http://www.amazon.com/author/paulachenderson